D0742789

Compulsive Acts

Compulsive Acts

*A Psychiatrist's Tales of Ritual
and Obsession*

Elias Aboujaoude, MD

UNIVERSITY OF CALIFORNIA PRESS

Berkeley   Los Angeles   London

University of California Press, one of the most distinguished
university presses in the United States, enriches lives around
the world by advancing scholarship in the humanities, social
sciences, and natural sciences. Its activities are supported by
the UC Press Foundation and by philanthropic contributions from individuals and institutions. For more information, visit www.ucpress.edu.

University of California Press
Berkeley and Los Angeles, California

University of California Press, Ltd.
London, England

Library of Congress Cataloging-in-Publication Data

Aboujaoude, Elias.
    Compulsive acts : a psychiatrist's tales of ritual and
obsession / Elias Aboujaoude.
        p.   cm.
    Includes bibliographical references and index.
    ISBN: 978-0-520-25567-8 (cloth : alk. paper)
    1. Obsessive-compulsive disorder—Anecdotes.
2. Compulsive behavior—Anecdotes.   I. Title.   II. Title:
Psychiatrist's tales of ritual and obsession.
    [DNLM: 1. Obsessive-Compulsive Disorder—
psychology—Personal Narratives.   2. Obsessive-
Compulsive Disorder—psychology—Popular Works.
3. Professional-Patient Relations—Personal Narratives.
4. Professional-Patient Relations—Popular Works.
WM 176 A155c 2008]

    RC533.A25   2008
    616.85'227—dc22   2007027445

Manufactured in the United States of America

17 16 15 14 13 12 11 10 09 08
10 9 8 7 6 5 4 3 2 1

The paper used in this publication meets the minimum requirements of ANSI/NISO z39.48–1992 (R 1997) (*Permanence of
Paper*).

For the memory of Danielle T. Kormos

CONTENTS

PREFACE

It is a tempting cliché to say I write because I am a busy psychiatrist with a deep supply of interesting stories. But it would be more original—and more accurate—to say I am a psychiatrist because I have always written or, more precisely, because I have always wanted to write.

For as long as I can remember, narratives have swirled around me—it helps to come from a large Mediterranean family whose members have big personalities and intertwined lives. Most of these stories flowed linearly, according to the universal rules of character development and narrative progression. Others, however, defied logic and made little sense, so I looked, by becoming a psychiatrist, for either the tools that could help me connect the dots or the peaceful acceptance that there are behaviors that cannot be explained and stories that are not meant to be understood.

Yet, although storytelling has been an important part of my life for a long time, I have not until now written a book for a wide nonscientific audience. Lack of a suitable protagonist may help explain this. For better or worse, stories, like history, are written about outliers, people at the extremes of the bell-shaped curve. Most of the extraordinary characters I conjured up, however, left me wondering whether their oddity would make them inaccessible to the general reader—that is, until I thought of writing stories loosely based on patients I treated in my psychiatric specialty of obsessive-compulsive disorder (OCD) and behavioral addictions such as kleptomania, gambling, and Internet abuse. These patient-inspired tales possessed the universal, easy-to-relate-to dimension of human suffering. But these stories were also unique in that the rituals and behaviors they depicted were highly unusual and, if I may call them that, colorful. The suffering I saw in these patients, combined with the peculiarity of the symptoms causing it, struck me as a worthy subject for my writing, and convinced me to finally stop *thinking* of myself as a writer and to actually become one.

This choice of subject also allowed me to describe some of the innovative research that our group at Stanford University has conducted over the past few years. Our research into previously little-studied topics like kleptomania and problematic Internet use has been published in peer-reviewed journals and widely covered in the media, often with a dose of sensationalism. Sharing our work with a lay audience and "setting the record straight" about what can and cannot be inferred from it provided me with additional motivation to pursue this subject.

But this book is not merely a disjointed collection of research anecdotes and clinical tales. Tying the individual stories together is the overarching theme of my own journey so far in psychiatry and the growth and learning that continue with every patient

I see, as well as the fascinating dramas unfolding over time among psychiatric clinic staff. Far more than a miscellany of memorable cases, then, this story has a beginning, a middle, and an end.

A work inspired by real patients is, however, a fraught affair, and it would be easy for it to end up causing more harm than good. I am referring especially to the possibility of violating a person's privacy. One way to avoid such a breach of trust would be to obtain the patient's informed consent and then freely tell the actual story, using initials in place of the full name. But there are at least two problems with this tactic. First, the patient is never the sole hero of the story. Even if the person agrees to having the story told, what about the long-suffering boyfriend or girlfriend who features so prominently in it, or the abusive parent whose behaviors weigh so heavily on the patient? If these supporting characters can potentially be recognized in the text, should I obtain their consent too? Where should I draw the line? Second, what if a patient has a change of heart about the story being made public as circumstances inevitably change? How would the person handle the fact that what has already been committed to paper cannot be withdrawn?

For all these reasons, it seemed to me that a safer approach would be to adhere to the *spirit* of the story, fictionalizing any identifying details to make the subject and other active players unrecognizable. And this is the path I chose to take. To that end, patient-specific characteristics such as name, gender, age, profession, family history, social background, symptoms, and treatment details have all been modified to varying degrees with an eye toward protecting confidentiality. In following this approach, I am adhering to a century-old tradition of privacy-conscious medical writing that has enriched both medicine and literature.

Moreover, I wanted from my book an opportunity to teach, so I wove medical data into each story, both to inform the narrative and to educate the reader. However, because I did not intend to write a book that was for patients or clinicians exclusively, I kept this information at a level accessible to a general audience. That is why the selective data presented here should not be viewed as a comprehensive guide to diagnosis or treatment, but rather as an instructional tool. Readers interested in more detailed information about the disorders in question are invited to consult the bibliography.

This educational aspect is all the more meaningful to me because this book is a tribute to my teacher, Danielle T. Kormos. To her memory I owe any writer in me, and other potentially saving graces. This is a book and a memorial.

Compulsive Acts

Psychiatry by the Dumpster

George was special from day one. I can still remember Dawn, my clinic clerk, paging me at 1:45 P.M., three quarters of an hour after his first scheduled appointment, to warn me: "Oh, Dr. A., you're gonna love this one!"

"Please don't tell me the patient just showed up," I said. "How am I supposed to do a full intake in the remaining fifteen minutes?"

"I know," Dawn answered, "but I couldn't just let him go. I don't know what to say, but he's—how should I put it?—he has his reasons for being late . . . He's special, even by our standards in this clinic, and even after nine years of doing this! I had to go out into the parking lot to check him in. That should give you an idea . . .

"You went to the parking lot to check him in?" I asked. "Outside?"

"Yes, outside," Dawn answered. "He can't come in, he says. Our door isn't wide enough for him."

"Our door isn't wide enough?" I queried, wondering whether I was the right doctor for this patient. "Did he mistake us for the gastric bypass clinic? How heavy is he?"

"Oh, he's not heavy at all," Dawn answered. "In fact, his wife tells me he hasn't eaten in a few days. He's just . . . I don't know . . . Something about his nose . . . He won't let anyone or anything close to it . . . He was so worried about his nose, he wouldn't even get into the car this morning."

"How did he make it to our clinic, then?" I asked. "I thought he lived in Belmont. That's fifteen miles away."

"He does," Dawn said. "He walked here. His wife drove, but George walked."

"He walked?" I asked in disbelief. "All the way from Belmont?"

"All the way from Belmont," Dawn repeated. "That's why I can't simply send him back and ask him to reschedule. Anyway, he *is* checked in now and waiting for you over in the far corner of the parking lot, exactly three feet from the dumpster, where, I might add, his wife spotted your old, squeaky office table and asked me to help her pull it out and put it in her trunk. I'm no doctor, but she's not right, either . . . What use could she possibly have for that table? Anyway, what would you like me to do now?"

"Well, I guess my only choice is to come right down," I said. "Meet me by the dumpster."

"OK, just remember not to get too close!" Dawn warned. "You might frighten him. And by the way, your two o'clock is here, too."

"Great! Is my two o'clock at least waiting in the waiting room?" I asked.

"Yes, she is," Dawn answered. "And I told her it was going to be a long wait . . ."

I walked toward Dawn, who was standing in the far corner of the parking lot. Nearby, in a vacant handicap spot by our recycling dumpster, stood George. In the adjacent spot, having managed with Dawn's help to squeeze my old filing cabinet into her trunk, stood his wife, now trying unsuccessfully to push the trunk door shut.

George was a lean twenty-something, with wide green eyes and a sunburned face and neck, probably from having walked a very long distance in the midday sun to come to my office. His grooming and hygiene left something to be desired, and his dirty fingernails and caked hair indicated more than just the wear and tear of one day's walkathon.

His wife started the conversation. "Dr. A., thank you for coming out here to see us," she said, still intent on shutting the trunk, despite one leg of my old office table clearly sticking out. "I know this is not standard practice, but it's very difficult to get him through doors anymore. I read up on obsessive-compulsive disorder, so I know how to diagnose it. Heck, I may even have a touch of it myself . . . We're here because we were told you were a specialist in OCD. It's urgent, Doctor! Things have gotten completely out of control since it's grown to three feet. *Three whole feet!*"

I was intrigued by the three feet but realized that I had not yet introduced myself to George. However, before I could formally do that, George preempted my handshake.

"I don't mean to be rude, Doctor," he said apologetically, "but please don't stick your hand out. I can't do handshakes."

"That's OK, I understand," I said. "I'm pleased to meet you anyway. Your wife just mentioned that 'it's grown to three feet.' What is it that has grown to three feet, George?"

"The radius around his nose," his wife answered, the quiver in her voice betraying her anxiety. "He needs that much clear space around his nose at all times. In the good old days, it used to be that nothing could come within a foot of his nose, and we could joke about it. But when the radius grew to two feet, it was anything but funny, and we started needing to make lifestyle modifications: having to sit alone in the backseat of the car, trying to sleep standing up like a horse, not to mention—if I may go there in your parking lot—the challenging sex . . ."

I could see Dawn's face tense up at the idea of "going there." The sexual comment was clearly in poor taste for her and went against deeply ingrained prohibitions on discussing private sexual matters even in clinical conversations—that is, if you can really call a parking lot discussion a "clinical conversation." Dawn soon found an outlet for her anxiety, however: she strode over to the trunk, broke off the old table's leg, threw it inside, and snapped the trunk closed with a satisfying thud.

The sound of the trunk shutting and the thought of securing the old cabinet for her home also dissipated George's wife's anxiety, and a relieved smile made its way to her face.

"But then," she continued, more at ease, "even two feet weren't enough. It had to grow to three feet, and at three feet, it has been, well, impossible to accommodate!"

Steering the conversation back to the principal patient, I asked, "How long has this been a problem for you, George?"

"Oh ever since . . . I don't know . . . It sort of crept up on me," he answered.

"Ever since his brother died," his wife interjected.

"When did that happen?" I asked.

"Two years ago," George answered. "He died in a skiing accident."

"I'm very sorry to hear that," I replied.

If sex had been difficult to discuss in the parking lot, death would have been even more so, so I asked George, "I know this is hard for you, but can you try once more to come up to my office so we can continue this important conversation in private?"

"I can't. I'm sorry," George answered, cautiously shaking his head. "Doorways are difficult for me. Hallways are challenging. And elevators are out of the question."

"Nothing personal, Doctor," George's wife added. "His father was visiting from Europe, where he lives, last month. We hadn't seen him in two years. Well, George wouldn't even give him a hug! All he could do was wave hi from a safe distance when he arrived at our house and wave goodbye when we dropped him off at the airport."

Seeing that the entire first meeting would probably have to be conducted outside, I wanted to make myself more comfortable. I went over to his wife's car to lean against the door, moving only slightly in George's direction. George responded briskly, stretching his arms out and twirling in a 360-degree circle, his arms fully extended. The move resembled a disc rotating on its axis; its purpose, I surmised, was to make sure the required radius of safety was not violated by my sudden movement and that I did not put his nose in any danger.

Sensing that I may have inadvertently increased George's anxiety, I tried to give him a little break by addressing my next question to his wife.

"You said you might have a touch of OCD, too," I said. "Tell me about it."

"Well, it's really just a touch," she said. "Nothing like this! I don't worry about injuring my nose, although I should! I broke it twice already, once in a car accident and once in a diving injury. My OCD, if we may call it that, actually makes sense . . . It's about making sure I don't run out of important things. 'What if I need it one day?' I always ask myself when I consider, or George makes me consider, throwing something out. And this simple question is usually enough to make me save the item, whatever it is. You can understand, then, how I built up my collection of pots and pans and cooking magazines and the tables I hope to stack them on. Did I mention cooking magazines? That is probably my biggest weakness!"

"Indeed," George agreed, gently nodding his head in agreement. "She has so many cooking magazines all over the kitchen, she can't make it to the stove to cook!" he added with a smile.

"That's right," his wife agreed. "I honestly can't remember the last time I cooked a meal for this poor man."

"But despite the mess in the kitchen," she continued, "we still eat well—or ate well, I should say—until his symptoms began. When he was at one foot, he couldn't use utensils, so I would buy him pizza, which he ate alone in his office. We lived on pizza for months because it didn't require a fork and knife. I would ask him, 'George, how come the pointy end of a pizza wedge is OK, but you can't use a knife and fork?' and he would say that something about metal approaching his nose was much scarier than the pointy end of the pizza wedge. Well, I thought it was kind of tragic, especially for someone who loved to eat and appreciated food so much. But oh, how I miss those days now! You see, when the radius grew to two feet, he couldn't even eat pizza, so he started insisting on soups and fluids, served in plastic bowls without a spoon. Later, when the radius grew to three feet, he started avoiding coming home altogether. He thought it was too much of a hazard, with all my stacks of cooking magazines and other stuff strewn all over the house. He didn't want to fall and hurt his nose, he said. So now he rents a studio nearby and eats—oh, I don't know what he eats, or *if* he eats . . . Look at how thin he's gotten!"

George did appear thin, but more than his low weight, it was his disheveled appearance that marked him as unhealthy, so I asked him, "What about basic activities of daily living besides eating? Toileting and hygiene, for instance?"

"This is really embarrassing, Doctor," George answered, looking down and away from me. "I can't shower anymore. I feel the showerhead is about to attack me. We even had a plumber come in to replace it. He said he would have to install the showerhead in our neighbors' kitchen if he adhered to my specifications of how far it should be from my head when I'm standing in the tub! I know it's crazy, Doctor, but I really can't help worrying about it."

"Worrying about things that don't make sense and constantly checking to make sure one is safe are common symptoms in OCD," I said. "It doesn't mean you're crazy. It means you have OCD, and that is only a small part of who you are. The good news is that for many patients OCD is quite responsive to treatment, so I'm glad you made the decision to come here today."

It is important during a first psychiatric meeting to try to get a fuller sense of the patient than his symptoms alone, so I inquired about George's hobbies and work experience next. Unfortunately, the conversation always came back to OCD. "What do you enjoy doing in your free time?" I asked. "Tell me more about the part of you that doesn't have OCD."

"Well, I used to sing in church," George answered, "but I've had to give that up, too. The idea of getting a microphone close to my nose is enough to make me mute with anxiety!"

"How about work, George?" I asked.

"I used to work in a large advertising firm," he answered. "I had to give that up, too. My cubicle got too small for my nose . . ." George smiled at the visual—an expanding nose in a shrinking cubicle—and I smiled, too, appreciating this young man's stubborn sense of humor, still evident despite the obvious stress he was under.

But many pieces of George's life and history were still unknown to me, and I could feel a hundred questions racing through my mind, all begging to be asked. By that point, though, I was very late for my two o'clock appointment, who was still patiently waiting for me, so I left George and his wife in the parking lot after getting their promise to return the following day so we could continue our "first meeting."

I did not leave them alone, though. I left them with Dawn, hoping that her powers of persuasion would be sufficient to get George inside the car.

"If I can get that old oversized table into your wife's trunk and manage to shut the door, I can get you into the car, too," she said to George as I walked away. As I overheard her ordering George's wife to open the sunroof, I cringed at the thought of what she might have in mind for George's trip home . . .

<hr />

We all have our peculiar habits and bizarre superstitions, but most of us don't suffer from OCD. Obsessive-compulsive disorder, the clinical condition, afflicts 1 to 2 percent of the population, and males and females are about equally likely to get it. For most sufferers, OCD is a chronic problem that will continue to negatively impact their lives, although the intensity of their symptoms may vary over time.

The fourth edition of the *Diagnostic and Statistical Manual*, or DSM-IV, the "bible" used by mental health professionals for diagnosing mental illness, defines OCD as the presence of obsessions *or* compulsions. To be clinically meaningful and meet DSM-IV requirements for a psychiatric diagnosis, the obsessions or compulsions must take up at least one hour daily and interfere substantially in the person's life. The DSM-IV criteria for diagnosing OCD are listed in on page 10.

Typically, OCD includes both obsessions *and* compulsions. Obsessions are unwanted thoughts, images, or impulses that come into the patient's mind in a repetitive way and that the patient experiences as bothersome. Common obsessions in OCD include contamination fears, such as fear of catching an infection or fear of pollution; "pathological doubt," especially about whether safety checks at home or in the car have been performed; symmetry obsessions, like the need to preserve things in perfect order; "somatic" obsessions about particular body parts or body functions, such as unjustified worries about one's nose or fear of fecal incontinence; and disturbing thoughts of a blasphemous or incestuous nature, as might be seen in a patient with no history of, or desire for, incestuous relationships, who has distressing mental images about having sex with a parent.

Compulsions are rituals performed by the person with OCD to neutralize the obsessions and reduce the anxiety they cause. Common compulsions include frequent checking of doors,

A. The presence of either obsessions or compulsions.
   Obsessions are defined by (1), (2), (3), and (4):

   1. recurrent thoughts, impulses, or images that are experienced as intrusive or unacceptable;

   2. the thoughts, impulses, or images are not simply excessive worries about real-life problems;

   3. the person attempts to ignore or suppress these thoughts, impulses, or images or to neutralize them by other thoughts or actions;

   4. the person recognizes that these thoughts, impulses, or images are the product of his own mind.

   Compulsions are defined by (1) and (2):

   1. repetitive behaviors or mental acts that the person feels compelled to perform in response to an obsession or to satisfy rigid, self-imposed rules;

   2. the behaviors or mental acts aim at reducing anxiety but are not logically connected to the source of anxiety or are excessive.

B. The person recognizes that these obsessions or compulsions are excessive or unreasonable.

C. The obsessions or compulsions cause distress and disability, and take up more than an hour daily.

D. The obsessions or compulsions are not better explained by another mental illness (e.g., are not limited to preoccupations with weight in a patient who has anorexia nervosa).

E. The symptoms are not due to substance use or a medical condition.

Source: Adapted from the *Diagnostic and Statistical Manual of Mental Disorders*, 4th ed. Washington, DC: American Psychiatric Press, 1994.

windows, stoves, car locks, or body parts; excessive cleaning, either of one's body or one's environment; hoarding of useless items in case they are needed in the future; and a need to repeatedly ask for reassurance or to confess perceived mistakes. Compulsions need not be observable behaviors and can be *mental* acts that the person performs, such as praying in rigid, preset ways, counting in silence up to a predefined number, or repeating certain words or sentences to oneself in fixed patterns "until it feels right."

Some compulsions cluster naturally with particular obsessions. For instance, excessive cleaning or hand-washing (the compulsion) often goes with contamination fears (the obsession), and frequent checking (the compulsion) often goes with pathological doubt (the obsession). Other obsession-compulsion pairs are not related in any "rational" way. For example, Sean, a pleasant young athlete I see in my clinic, experiences obsessive incestuous thoughts involving his sister. He is absolutely disgusted by these thoughts and has never had any desire or intention to act on them. For Sean, the compulsion that helps neutralize the anxiety accompanying this obsession consists of tapping his inner thigh five times every time the thought intrudes on his mind.

Of all compulsions, excessive checking is the most common and is seen in over 60 percent of people with OCD. Some checking compulsions take the form of exaggerated everyday behaviors that in normal individuals are automatically and quickly performed—examples include checking to make sure the doors are locked or that one did not accidentally hit a passerby while backing out of the driveway. A person with OCD, however, may spend several hours a day checking and rechecking, often in complex, uncompromising patterns.

The following scenario from a patient with OCD whom I treat for checking compulsions is representative. Before he can leave for work in the morning, Tim has to feel secure that the stove in his kitchen is turned off. His ritual demands that he check each knob five times, waiting sixty seconds every time with his hand on the knob to make sure it is in the "off" position. Given that his stove has four knobs, it takes Tim twenty minutes to complete this ritual before he can leave the house or, if he is going through a bad OCD period, before he can move on to other checking rituals, such as making sure the doors and windows are locked, the faucets in the bathroom are not leaking, the irrigation system in the garden is turned off, and the drains on the roof are not clogged.

Still, other checking rituals in OCD are much more unusual than Tim's. Two patients I treated come immediately to mind: Stephanie, who had to check that her left arm was still attached to her body by holding it inside her right hand and focusing intensely on it; and Paul, who, before allowing any piece of paper to leave his house, had to meticulously read and then shred it, "on the off chance I wrote my social security number on it by mistake."

But if their behaviors appeared bizarre to people around them, they also seemed strange to Stephanie and Paul themselves. People with OCD are usually well aware of how nonsensical their symptoms are and are often the first to describe them as "silly," "embarrassing," or "crazy." In Stephanie's case, when her husband tried to reassure her that her left arm was fine, her typical answer was, "Of course I know my left arm is fine. I'm perfectly healthy, physically. I just can't help checking to be sure." For Paul, when I asked him how he did not seem to worry about inadvertently writing his social security number down at work, he quickly answered, "I honestly can't explain why it doesn't bother me at work. I recycle papers there all the time without thinking twice about it. I even gave away my office shredder to a coworker! This doesn't make sense to me, either."

Still, in the most severe OCD cases, patients may lose such rational perspective on their illness and start thinking that their obsessions and compulsions make sense and are justified. A good example is Jeff, a patient I treated for irrational fears around catching the cold virus. Jeff fully believed that turning the closest light switch on and off ten times after shaking hands with people somehow boosted his immune system and protected him from getting a cold. Such OCD cases take on an almost psychotic dimension because the patient's reality-testing seems impaired. For that reason such a patient tends to be more difficult to treat—unfortunately, Jeff has been in therapy and on various combinations of medications for many years without any sustained improvement in his symptoms.

For our meeting the following day, George again walked from his apartment to my clinic. With much encouragement from his wife and Dawn, however, George was able to pass through the building's doors and climb the stairs to the clinic area, after performing a checking regimen that required a whole hour to complete: with each step he took from the building's main door to my office, George would make a 360-degree turn on his feet, his arms outstretched to clear the space around him. Dawn led his wife to the waiting room so I could meet with George privately.

Once inside my office, George used one hand to move a heavy wooden armchair from one corner of the room to the center, using the other hand as a protective shield for his nose in case he moved the chair too close to his face. He then very cautiously sat in the chair. As he performed this ritual, I found myself rolling my chair back into the corner to give him additional security.

"Why me?" was his first question.

"I wish I had a satisfactory answer for you," I said, "but, like so many other psychiatric and medical illnesses we see, we are much better at treating disease than at knowing exactly why a particular person develops a particular symptom."

"Did I somehow catch it from her?" he asked, referring to his wife but appearing suspicious about the premise of his question, as though he knew beforehand that the answer would be no. "But I don't hoard," he quickly added. "In fact, I'm the anti-hoarder."

"You cannot 'catch' OCD that way, George," I said. "You might have a genetic vulnerability to developing OCD if you had a close blood relative with it. However, even when OCD does cluster in families, its symptoms can vary greatly among family members."

"Well, I don't have any biological relatives with it, as far as I know," George quickly said.

"Speaking of catching things," I said, "do you spend a lot of time worrying about contamination or pollution? How about frequent checking that doesn't involve your nose? Any excessive cleaning, counting, touching, arranging, or worrying about other body parts besides your nose, now or in the past?"

"Never," George answered. "Other than this preoccupation with my nose, I've always been a pretty laid-back, relaxed guy."

"Do you worry that your nose may be weak or somehow deformed and in need of protection?" I asked. "Do you think it looks abnormal?"

"No, I think my nose looks just fine as it is now," George replied. "I'm very happy with it. I just want to keep it that way!"

"Do you have any reason to worry that it might not stay that way?" I asked. "Are you prone to accidents, for example? Have you ever seriously injured your nose or any other body part before?"

"Not really," George answered. "I've always been a cautious choirboy and high school debater kind of guy rather than the contact sports type."

After ascertaining that it was not the memory of some old physical trauma that made George worry about hurting himself, I wondered about a trauma he might have witnessed involving someone else, or even an emotional trauma. Thinking back to our first meeting, when his wife related the onset of George's OCD symptoms to losing his brother in a skiing accident two years ago, I said, "Tell me about your brother, George. Were you close?"

"Yes, very," George answered, looking down and away. "I was supposed to go with him on his skiing trip, but a choir event kept me back."

"I'm sorry to hear about what happened to him," I said. "Is it true that your OCD symptoms began shortly thereafter?"

"As I said, it sort of crept up on me," he answered, "but I would say sometime around then I started frequently checking my nose in the mirror to make sure it was OK."

The striking coincidence between the onset of George's OCD symptoms and the loss of his brother is rich in meaning and symbolism. It is relatively common for patients with OCD to experience their first symptoms or to relapse after a symptom-free period as a function of external stress. But beyond that, were George's specific symptoms somehow determined by the nature of the stress? Could the unexpected loss of a young, healthy brother to a fatal accident have made George overly vigilant about his own environment, in a desperate attempt to prevent a similar tragedy from happening to him?

However, before I could expand further on this hypothesis, we heard a light knock on the door. George's wife then cautiously walked in, careful not to swing the door fully open in a way that might disturb George, who was still sitting in a chair in the center of the room. She carefully deposited an oversized bag on the floor against the wall, then stood practically stuck to the wall.

"I thought I had given you enough time alone and was burning to ask you some questions about my role in George's treatment," she said. "For example, I feel sometimes like I'm colluding with him and making things worse, like when I agreed to unhinge and remove the French doors between the dining room and the living room to make the passageway safer for his nose. Should I have just said no and expected George to deal with the anxiety of navigating the doorway? Did I do more harm than good by giving in to his OCD?"

"You raise a very good question," I said. "It's a difficult balance that you're being asked to strike. On the one hand, it's a natural instinct to help your husband when he asks for it, but on the other hand, you know that giving in to his OCD can perpetuate his symptoms and allow him to avoid addressing them. In my opinion, the best way to handle this is to try to accommodate severe OCD fears that, if not allayed, would paralyze him. However, you should try to avoid giving in to lesser fears you think he can handle on his own. There's a way to do this that teaches him how to work through his anxiety and be more independent."

As I tried to explain to George's wife her role in treating her husband's OCD symptoms, I couldn't help but think of a possible indirect role she might have played in *causing* them. From my previous conversations with George about his wife and what I witnessed in the parking lot when she rescued a useless old table from the dumpster and took it home, it was clear that George's wife also suffered from a form of OCD, which manifested itself primarily in hoarding behavior. Could her collections of useless objects and magazines cluttering the house be even more obstructive to George than the French doors in her example? Would another way to understand George's specific symptom and his need for space be as an unconscious retaliation against his wife for the hoarding that had severely cluttered their lives? By becoming so debilitated by objects that stick out and eventually having to leave the house because of it, was George signaling to his wife his distress over the state of the house and her inability to fully acknowledge her own illness and get treatment for it? A Freudian psychiatrist might read in George's symptoms—and expose to him in the course of therapy—the following unconscious message to his wife: it's time for you to give the house a cleaning, to admit that you have OCD yourself, and to do something about it.

It was, of course, a delicate dance. While I wanted to try to point out features of George's wife's behavior that might have promoted and contributed to her husband's symptoms, I could not afford to forget that George, not his wife, was my patient. It wasn't my role to diagnose or treat her, especially since she was only willing to accept that she had a "touch" of OCD. Still, I would have liked to gently explain to her the possible interplay between her "touch" of OCD and her husband's full-blown condition, but another knock on my door, followed by Dawn's entry, interrupted me.

Dawn was very careful not to swing the door fully open. Once inside, she also positioned herself against the wall, adding to the drama of the "set." As it now stood, the configuration of bodies and furniture in my office was as follows: George in his chair in the exact center of the room, me in mine tucked in the far corner opposite the door, George's wife plastered against the wall on one side of the door, and Dawn adopting the same position on the other. Between the two women, also stuck to the wall, was George's wife's oversized bag.

"I'm not just being unreasonable because I haven't eaten all day," Dawn said, referring to the annual Lent fast she had just begun, "but we have a problem on our hands, and we'd better address this now." Then, looking alternately at George's wife and the bag on the floor, she pronounced, "You cannot do that. I saw you. You cannot take the cooking magazines from our waiting room. What's in the dumpster outside is fair game, but not what's inside the building! We can help you if you need help, but you cannot be taking our magazines, especially since we work hard to keep our reading material up to date compared to other clinics!"

An uncomfortable silence descended on the room, which George finally tried to break with an attempt at humor: "I guess you have kleptomania on top of hoarding, my dear," he said, gently shaking his head and chuckling briefly.

But there was nothing humorous in any of this for his wife. Her face turned deep red, and she tried hard to avoid the other three sets of eyes in the room. Seeing how much embarrassment she had caused, Dawn quickly sought to defuse the situation: "But I promise to save any *old* issues for you if you want!"

⁂

Dawn, née Aurora, is much more to our clinic than her clerical title would suggest. Our schedule is like a symphony of which she is the masterful conductor. She makes sure records are up to date, orders are placed before supplies run out, and unpleasant communications with insurance companies are handled with minimal doctor involvement if at all possible. But, far more than her unquestionable administrative skills, it is Dawn's unique style and her compelling story that make her so indispensable to our clinic.

Coming in for a psychiatric evaluation, especially if it's a patient's first contact with the mental health system, can be a traumatic experience. With Dawn on the front lines handling phone calls and check-ins, the patient is guaranteed to receive caring, experienced service that conveys a you-don't-need-to-worry-I've-seen-it-all-before attitude that is both blasé and oddly comforting. And on the rare occasions when she comes across as abrasive or demanding, as she did with George's wife on the couple's second appointment, the deep reserve of trust and respect that the patient, his family, and of course the doctor have for her allows us to see her behavior as a manifestation of "tough love" ultimately in the patient's and the clinic's best interest rather than as an intentional breach or an unforgivable faux pas. And so we put up with Dawn operating sometimes on the peripheries of what is sensitive or totally appropriate because we're convinced that patients will ultimately be better off for it, and the clinic will run more smoothly as a result.

But if tough love is her modus operandi at work, when it comes to Hector, her husband of fifteen years, Dawn is all love, all the time, without any toughness. Ever since the couple, then in their early twenties, emigrated from Mexico some twelve years ago, they have been inspiring in their commitment to each other and their pursuit of what one might still call the American dream:

happiness, self-improvement, and material comfort for themselves and their children.

In people observing Dawn and Hector's hard work and enthusiasm for their new life, they rekindle the optimistic belief in America as the land of possibilities. Years ago, for example, she decided to change her name from Aurora to Dawn to mark the English-only policy she instituted at home to help her girls learn English and fully integrate at school. More recently, Hector took what might be considered the quintessential new American job— an unpaid clerical position with a new Internet start-up company in exchange for stock options that might eventually translate into cash if the company succeeds; as a result, Dawn, now the sole breadwinner, has had to take all the overtime hours she could to supplement the family's income.

Through it all, Dawn has handled her immigrant family's struggle to enter the U.S. middle class with dignity, hope, and remarkable resilience. But on those rare days when the pressures of life combined with clinic stress get to her, Dawn can always count on one of her well-meaning, usually also foreign-born fellow clerks to lend an ear and to remind her how it could all be so much worse . . . How, for instance, one of her girls could be afflicted with severe OCD, or how she and her family could still be living in poverty in Mexico City, or both!

▒∴▒ ▭ ▒∴▒

OCD does sometimes seem like a natural disaster visited on the unlucky. To explain why some people develop this illness, we have to borrow information from neurobiology as well as various schools of psychology. There is little debate that OCD, like many other psychiatric conditions, has biological roots. Brains of patients with OCD actually look different when scanned, both in the overall size of certain brain regions and in the higher blood flow and metabolic activity seen. More intriguingly, successful treatment of OCD symptoms with medications or therapy seems to correct these differences so brain patterns become indistinguishable from what you see in people without OCD. Such measurable differences in parts of the OCD patient's brain point strongly to at least a partly biological explanation for the disorder.

So does what is happening at the level of the neurons, the individual brain cells that make up the brain centers. Serotonin, a neurotransmitter—that is, a naturally occurring chemical substance that neurons use to communicate with each other—seems to play a crucial role in OCD. The best evidence for a serotonin link to OCD is that all antidepressants that work by increasing the level of serotonin in the brain seem to help OCD, whereas those that work through other neurotransmitters usually do not. Recently, medical interest has shifted to another neurotransmitter, glutamate, which is present in higher concentrations in some parts of the brain in people with OCD and which seems to decrease to normal levels after successful treatment with medication.

However, one central question remains: are such biological features—the measurable differences in some regions of the brain, the low serotonin, and the high glutamate—present at the origins of OCD, somehow causing it, or are they the downstream effects of having suffered from this illness? These findings in the brains of patients with OCD could still turn out to be the *result* of a biological transformation the disease itself inflicts on the brain, not unlike, for instance, chronic depression, which has been shown to lead over time to a visible shrinking of the hippocampus, a region of the brain that is important in memory storage and processing.

Another important argument in support of the biological roots of OCD is the genetic link. The percentage of identical twins in which both individuals have OCD is consistently higher than that of fraternal twins. Given that the environmental influences are the same among identical and fraternal twins but that only identical twins share the same genetic material, an argument has been made for the importance of "nature" over "nurture" in the development of OCD.

Nature or biology, however, can offer only part of the answer. Various schools of psychology have also tried to explain OCD. The oldest, most colorful, and probably most discredited psychological explanation is the model offered by Freudian psychoanalysis. In his book *Notes upon a Case of Obsessional Neurosis*, first published in 1909, Sigmund Freud describes Ernst Lanzer, or Rat Man, a young university-educated man with intrusive thoughts of seeing and touching nude girls (the obsession) and an associated fear that, if he did not control these impulses, he would somehow cause significant harm to happen to his father. Specifically, he feared that his father would be subjected to a particularly cruel form of torture: having rats burrow into his anus while he was tied up—hence the pseudonym Rat Man. Rat Man developed elaborate rituals (the compulsion) around these thoughts to help reduce his anxiety and ward off the impending evil. Freud, through an analysis of the patient's sexual development, saw Rat Man's symptoms as manifestations of horror and guilt over some early, prohibited sexual fantasies he had as a child that were now stored in the unconscious mind, surfacing in the form of disturbing obsessions and waiting to be processed with the help of psychoanalysis.

Psychoanalytic exploration then aims at uncovering the repressed fear at the basis of these symptoms and resolving the underlying conflicts. According to this theory, such uncovering, by making the unconscious conscious, would lead to recovery from OCD. After analyzing Rat Man for one year using this approach, Freud pronounced his patient cured. However, not much is known about the long-term success of Freud's intervention: Ernst Lanzer died in the fields of World War I.

Evolutionary psychology approaches the OCD problem through the Darwinian lens of natural selection based on overall fitness for survival. One can see how it might be helpful for our species to possess the ability to generate anxiety-provoking obsessions while in a safe environment because these can help the brain to learn and practice risk avoidance behaviors; should the organism then be faced with a real threat from the environment, this "safety training" could serve as a good template to follow. It is intriguing to note, for instance, how often the elaborate obsessions and compulsions seen in OCD can be reduced to the common themes of safety and self-preservation: washing protects against disease, hoarding food protects against famine, and frequent checking of the environment keeps us out of harm's way. In the individual with OCD, it is thought, these basically good, potentially life-saving traits are somehow disinhibited and allowed to go unchecked, so to speak.

George did not wish to approach his OCD as a novel with villains and victims. He didn't see a very convincing connection between his brother's untimely death or his wife's hoarding problem on the one hand and the onset of his OCD symptoms or the nature of these symptoms on the other. The most he would agree to was that the overall level of stress that his brother's death and his wife's condition had caused him somehow made his OCD vulnerability, which had already been there, finally express itself.

And I basically agreed. I felt that pursuing these impossible-to-prove associations too forcefully, against George's stated preference, could paradoxically lead him to attribute meaning to symptoms that he saw as essentially meaningless and indefensible. Following a psychoanalytic approach that imbued symptoms with a rational dimension through cause-and-effect linkages ran the risk of making them meaningful, and hence perhaps worthy of holding on to.

Instead, the idea of OCD as a chemical imbalance that happens for reasons we do not fully understand is what resonated with George, in part because it removed the blame: it was no longer a personal failing on his part, nor was it his brother's or wife's fault. He had researched the serotonin hypothesis for OCD and favored a chemical solution to what he viewed as essentially a chemical problem.

"So what SSRI are you starting me on?" George asked at the beginning of our third meeting, before I had fully discussed pharmacological treatments with him.

"I'm very impressed," I said. "It looks like you've done your homework. Do you know how these medications work?"

"Something about serotonin," George answered.

"Indeed," I said. "Selective serotonin reuptake inhibitors, or SSRIs, work by increasing levels of serotonin in the brain."

"What's the likelihood of them working?" he wanted to know.

"The response rate is around 50 to 60 percent, and it seems similar across all SSRIs," I told him.

"So how do you decide which one to give, then?" he asked.

"Well, I decide in part based on any previous medication trials you may have had," I explained. "It's also important to consider what else you may be taking currently, because drugs can interact with each other. If you have family members with OCD, we should look at what medications they responded to, since there seems to be a genetic component to response, just like there's a genetic component to having OCD."

"Well, I've never been treated for OCD before," George said. "I don't take any other meds, and I have no blood relatives with OCD to help guide us. So it's a clean slate!"

"Well, this leaves us with side-effect profiles to help us decide," I suggested. "The most likely side effect to this class of medications in a healthy young man would probably be sexual."

"I cannot even hug my wife, let alone think of having sex." George answered, smiling slightly at the irony. "Sexual side effects are simply not an issue for me right now."

"Well, let's start Zoloft, then," I said. "It's relatively clean and well tolerated. As with all SSRIs, though, when taking them for OCD, you have to wait up to ten weeks for a response. The starting dose is usually 50 mg daily, and our target will be 100 to 200 mgs, if we're not limited by side effects."

⚅⚁⚅

Although first developed as antidepressants, selective serotonin reuptake inhibitors (SSRIs) have been shown to be effective in several anxiety disorders, including OCD. In double-blind placebo-controlled research studies, neither the investigators conducting the study nor the subjects participating in it know who is taking an active drug and who is taking an identical-looking sugar pill, or placebo. These studies are considered the gold standard for establishing a drug's efficacy, and all six SSRIs currently available in the United States have passed the double-blind test, with at least one large study yielding positive results. Hence, fluvoxamine (Luvox), fluoxetine (Prozac), sertraline (Zoloft), paroxetine (Paxil), citalopram (Celexa), and escitalopram (Lexapro) can all be considered reasonable first-line pharmacological treatments for OCD, although not all have been approved by the U.S. Food and Drug Administration (FDA) for that purpose. (It is not uncommon for medications to be effective in, and prescribed for, conditions for which they do not carry FDA approval.)

Looking at these studies as a group, we can draw several conclusions useful in guiding treatment. First, about 50 to 60 percent of patients with OCD respond to treatment with an SSRI. Also, higher doses of the SSRI are usually required to treat OCD than what is generally needed for depression, and the length of treatment before a response is seen is generally longer (about ten weeks for OCD compared to about four weeks for depression). Moreover, despite the fact that all SSRIs work by raising serotonin levels in the brain, patients with OCD who do not respond to one SSRI still have a good chance of responding to another one. Finally, despite the high doses often required, these medications appear to be generally well tolerated. A discussion of second-line pharmacological treatments for OCD and of the many ways in which medications are combined is beyond the scope of this book.

Drugs alone, however, are often not sufficient to treat OCD and may lead to high relapse rates after they are discontinued, whereas therapy, it is argued, can teach the patient tools that last a lifetime. For many patients, combining medications with a form of therapy known as *cognitive behavioral therapy*, or CBT, offers the most relief. Unlike psychoanalysis, CBT has proved effective in well-designed studies. In CBT, the patient is asked to develop a hierarchy of feared OCD scenarios and is then exposed to gradually escalating situations over several therapy sessions, starting with the least feared and progressing through the list. For example, Craig, a thirty-something lawyer I treated for OCD, had a severe contamination obsession that prevented him from using the bathroom at the law firm where he worked. I started Craig's treatment by asking him to simply walk past the bathroom once daily for a week. After one week, I asked Craig to open the bathroom door once a day without going inside. The "homework" gradually became more demanding, requiring Craig to walk into the bathroom daily and use the sink, then the urinal, until finally I was able to ask him to confront the worst fear he listed on his hierarchy, namely, using the toilet. We addressed Craig's accompanying ritual of excessive hand-washing similarly, by gradually reducing the amount of time he was allowed to keep the water running.

And as I walked Craig through the hierarchy of feared situations, I encouraged him to "ride the anxiety wave," teaching him relaxation techniques like deep breathing and giving him copious reassurances that the more he faced the obsession and the more he avoided the ritual, the easier it would become for him to do so.

However, OCD symptoms are often so severe that the patient is unable to engage in meaningful therapy. Cognitive behavioral therapy is a collaborative approach that assumes a motivated patient willing and able to come into the therapist's office for what is usually an hourly session every week for several months. The therapist assigns homework that the patient is expected to complete between sessions and holds the patient accountable for failure to do so. Such work is impossible with patients who are difficult to engage or who cannot leave their house, drive a car, or come into a clinic building because of the severity of their OCD symptoms. So, when a patient's personality or the severity of symptoms precludes adequate cognitive behavioral therapy, medication should be started alone, with the option of incorporating therapy into the treatment once the patient improves and is better able to engage in therapy and tolerate its requirements.

In addition to being his prescribing doctor, I wanted to serve as George's therapist, and in many ways, George would have been an ideal candidate for therapy. A responsible and inquisitive young man, he seemed to have the youth and mental flexibility needed for change and the creativity and faith to see how the talking process can alter brain chemistry enough to effect this change. Using the cognitive behavioral model, I imagined myself assigning him homework and his reporting back to me on his weekly progress. I imagined focusing first on the basic tasks needed to meet some vital needs, such as food and hygiene. For instance, I would start by increasing his comfort level with eating utensils, while working on his fear of the showerhead. We could then move toward getting him back to work, perhaps part-time initially, maybe in an expanded cubicle. I would also try to help him gradually feel comfortable being intimate with his wife again—maybe have him move back into the house at first but sleep in a different room, then in the same room but on the floor, then in the same bed, then have him hold her hand, then hug her, then . . . But so much for my plans for therapy—it was impossible to get George to come in for the regular sessions needed to make it happen. The length of time it took him to work through his anxiety just to make it to his appointments caused him to miss several sessions and created an almost impossible therapy relationship.

George *was*, however, very committed to taking his medication. So instead of face-to-face weekly clinic meetings, I made the decision to treat him with the medication alone at first, and I monitored his progress and any side effects through phone contact every other week. I still fantasized, though, about the step-by-step therapy course I would take him through and thought that the strong doctor-patient alliance, of the kind that could be achieved only through intensive therapy, was indispensable for a successful outcome in his case. In my mind, it was a matter of when, not if, I would bring therapy to the aid of Zoloft.

But by our second phone contact after starting the medication (his fifth week on it), George's voice already sounded somehow significantly more resonant and self-assured. Could it be that my therapy intervention might not be needed after all?

"You sound clearer today, George," I commented. "Are you feeling better?"

"I am," George said. Then, sounding almost euphoric, he added, "But there's also a technical reason for why I sound better."

"A technical reason?" I asked. "What is it?"

"Well, I'm calling from home, which helps," he answered, "and I'm actually able to use the handset today! When I spoke with you before, I had to be on the speaker phone. I couldn't tolerate the handset so close to my nose."

"This is great, George," I exclaimed. "Did you have to push yourself to use the handset for our phone call today? How much of a struggle was it?"

"It really wasn't a struggle at all," George answered. "I just didn't think about it. It somehow didn't occur to me today that the handset would hurt my nose. I only realized after dialing your number that, oh my God, I'm actually holding the phone! My only explanation is that the Zoloft must be doing its thing already . . .

"I think you're right," I agreed. "I think we're seeing an early response. That's wonderful news that . . ."

"And I have more wonderful news for you," George interrupted. "I also had a real shower this morning for the first time in a long while. I feel fresh for a change."

"I'm sure that helps, too," I said. "How about another basic function, eating? Are you still afraid of utensils and solid foods and can only drink fluids?"

"I certainly can't handle pizza yet," George answered. "The wedge thing still bothers me, so do knives and forks, but the good news on that front is that I can tolerate spoons now! For some reason, I'm more comfortable with round forms approaching my nose than pointy edges. That's how I could eat a hamburger yesterday— a fat juicy one that tasted like the best burger I ever had!"

"It's so nice to see you come out of this, George," I said. "We're only at week five, so we can still expect more improvement over the next couple of weeks. As I told you, many patients don't get better until week ten or so."

"Let's up the dose anyway, Doc!" George suggested.

"Well, you're tolerating 50 mg pretty well, so let's go up to 100 mg and stay there for a while," I concurred. "Call me at the same time in two weeks, and we'll reassess."

But before I could let George go, I had to inquire about his wife's hoarding. I had decided that her behavior was contributing to my patient's symptoms by increasing the ambient stress in the household, so I felt justified inquiring into it.

"Before you go," I said, "can I ask you how your wife is doing with her hoarding these days? You said you moved back in, so I want to be optimistic and think that the house feels more hospitable to you. I realize it's not my place to treat her, but . . ."

"Funny you should ask!" George broke in. "You know, her mother who's a neat freak, her father who's a perfectionist in his own right, and I who worry about hurting my nose, all have for years been telling her to clean up the house but to no avail. Until, that is, your Dawn caught her in the act of stocking up! Well, I'm glad to report that your assistant's intervention is working where nothing else ever has! Maybe out of embarrassment over what happened, my wife has for the first time decided to confront her problem. She has finally agreed to hire a professional declutterer that her mom recommended, a very methodical woman with a stern old nun quality to her who will not take no for an answer when my wife refuses to let her throw something away—exactly what my wife needs! Well, 'Mother Superior,' as we started calling her, has already begun her journey into the heart of darkness that is our kitchen. The output so far, in case you're wondering? Fifteen boxes of cooking magazines, yellowed with age, not with extra virgin olive oil stains!"

Hoarding is defined as the acquisition and difficulty getting rid of worthless items. About 20 percent of patients with OCD have as their most prominent symptoms compulsive hoarding and obsessive fears of throwing out items that might be needed in the future. Items most commonly saved include magazines, newspapers, old clothing, mail (including junk mail), and lists of all kinds. Although such collecting can be problematic in all age groups, the elderly are especially vulnerable due to the real threat it can pose to their safety by causing falls, fires, and the inability to prepare food or adhere to medication regimens because of difficulty navigating their kitchens or finding their pills.

Hoarding appears to differ on several important fronts from more "classic" symptoms of OCD, such as contamination fears or excessive checking. This has caused experts to wonder whether hoarding is a distinct disorder altogether rather than simply a form of OCD. For instance, compared to other presentations of OCD, hoarding-type OCD is generally much less responsive to treatment, especially pharmacological interventions, and only mildly responsive to therapy. Furthermore, imaging studies of the brain have shown different rates of metabolic activity in some brain regions among hoarders compared to people who have OCD but do not hoard.

Semana Santa, or Holy Week, has always been a very special time of year for Dawn. It is the culmination of a process that begins on Ash Wednesday, when Dawn arrives earlier than usual for work after morning Mass, bearing an ashen cross imprinted on her forehead. This is the official beginning of the Lent season for her, a forty-day period leading up to Easter that she observes by completely avoiding meat and adhering, well, religiously, to a strict fasting regimen that starts at sunrise and ends at sunset every day.

Watching Dawn follow this Catholic ritual every year helps punctuate the calendar for the rest of the clinic staff too. Several national and international medical meetings happen in late spring because of the generally good travel weather. Dawn's fast, which usually falls sometime in April, is a good wake-up call, reminding us that conference deadlines are fast approaching and that by the time Dawn breaks her fast at the end of Lent, we should have ended our procrastination and finished writing up the research to be presented at these meetings. Otherwise it will be too late. So, indirectly, Dawn's annual fast is generally beneficial to the non-Catholics in the clinic as well, inspiring increased productivity on everyone's part. Perhaps because of this fringe benefit, we are more tolerant than we might otherwise be of the slight increase in irritability, which slowly builds up in Dawn through the day every day during Lent as her hunger pangs gradually worsen.

But Dawn's ascetic self-denial for forty long days only heightens the drama of what comes next: the ritual-heavy Semana Santa, or Holy Week, building up to Easter Sunday. Palm Sunday is the official start of Semana Santa, commemorating for Christians Jesus's entry into Jerusalem; in preparation, Dawn breaks off small branches from the dwarf palm tree in our parking lot and takes them home for decoration. Spy Wednesday comes a few days later and recalls Judas's spying on Jesus; Dawn commemorates that by leaving work early to go to Mass. The following day is Maundy Thursday, when the story of Jesus's Last Supper is retold; Dawn also marks it by leaving work early to go to Mass. Then comes Good Friday, recalling Christ's Crucifixion and burial; out of respect, Dawn wears all black that day and avoids makeup. Holy Saturday follows next, and, sometime between sundown on Holy Saturday and the morning of Easter Sunday, when Resurrection is celebrated, a Mass takes place that constitutes for Dawn the absolute liturgical highlight of her year—until the following year, that is, when the entire cycle is played out again.

Rituals are woven into the fabric of our daily lives. It seems as though rituals, performed automatically and according to inherited, rarely questioned recipes, are the glue that holds a group together, setting it aside from other groups—with different rituals—but also connecting it with past and future generations. In our remarkable willingness to partake in, and pass on, rituals like the Passover Seder, graduation ceremonies, burials, coronations, or the Thanksgiving menu, we express a built-in need for fixed behaviors that repeat themselves, unchanged, over time. This constancy comforts us and punctuates our lives, bringing us order, or *seder* in Hebrew. It is also a big part of what defines culture.

How, then, do the ritualistic behaviors we see in OCD fit into this generally positive function of rituals in our lives? Without getting into a moot discussion of how much is too much, we can safely start by saying that OCD rituals are excessive. But deeper than that, OCD rituals either become an end unto themselves or are performed in response to mounting anxiety. In other words, the elaborate, time-consuming rituals we see in OCD are bereft of the symbolism and meaning that something like a bar mitzvah celebration can command. Furthermore, OCD rituals tend to be self-generated. Unlike, say, Judaism's and Islam's proscription against eating pork, a tradition which practicing parents inculcate in their children and which can then become a lifelong connection with ancestors and faith, a patient with OCD who suddenly develops an irrational fear of eating chicken is acting largely independently and not sharing in a communal practice. In this case, ritual becomes an isolating oddity rather than a shared behavior that, although perhaps a bit peculiar to some observers, still fosters community and encourages engagement.

Exactly two weeks after our last phone contact, at the time of the scheduled call, instead of my phone ringing I heard an assertive knock on my door. It was George, only much cleaner than at our last face-to-face meeting some two months before. His wife stood next to him, her svelte frame curving slightly in George's direction under pressure from his arm, which he had wrapped tightly around her waist. The sight of the intimate-looking couple clearly indicated to me that the three-, two-, or even one-foot rule was no longer in effect—and that George was probably not having sexual side effects!

"What a nice surprise!" I said, addressing George. "You look great."

"Doesn't he now?" his wife beamed. "I have my husband back. He even drove us here!"

"*And* we have a gift for you," George said, handing me a wedge-shaped present wrapped in aluminum foil and smelling of pepperoni.

"You brought me pizza?" I asked, surprised and moved by this gesture.

"Yes," George answered. "I bet no patient has ever given you pizza before!"

"No, no patient ever has," I concurred. "This is a first indeed. Thank you."

"Well, pizza has been a recurring theme in our conversations," George explained, "and, in a way, it's the best measure of both how silly and how disabling my OCD was. All this makes it a fitting final thank-you gift."

"Well, I'm very touched, George," I said. "Thank you again."

"Wait!" his wife interjected, "It gets even better . . ."

"How much better can it get?" I asked, wondering what other pleasant surprises the couple had in store for me.

"It's homemade!" George exclaimed, elated at the thought of a home-cooked meal.

"You're able to use your stove again?" I almost gasped, looking at George's wife.

"I can indeed!" she said proudly, "and we have our declutterer, or 'Mother Superior,' to thank for it! I just have to make sure I maintain now. 'For each item that makes it into the sanctum of your home, an equal or larger item has to exit,' she ceremoniously warned me at our last meeting."

"In my experience, that is probably the best advice for hoarders and more likely to help than any medication or even therapy intervention," I agreed. "Your approach of having someone do the throwing for you while you deal with the anxiety this generates, and while you work on maintaining the result, is probably the way to go." Then, turning toward George, I said, "What *you* have to maintain, and probably for a while, is your medication."

"Oh, don't worry, Doc," George said. "I don't plan to stop it anytime soon." Then he added, half-jokingly, "But my wife has a burning question for you. It's been keeping her up at night!"

"What's your question?" I asked.

"Is it true, Doctor, that animals, too, can get OCD?" she asked, leaning in my direction and looking intently into my eyes as though she had indeed been burning to ask the question.

"And where did you hear of such a thing?" I queried.

"Well, a magazine I discovered behind the stove while cleaning the kitchen had an article saying that dogs, too, can get OCD," she said. "Apparently, they start cleaning and licking themselves, and they just can't stop! Some even get infections and die from it. And if all this was not shocking enough, the article talks about medications in the Zoloft family that can actually cure them! I had to hide the magazine and save it from 'Mother Superior,' of course. In case we ever have a dog with OCD, at least we'll know how to treat him!"

"And do you have a dog now?" I asked, trying to empathize with her worry but also quite amused by it.

"We have two," she answered.

"And do they have this problem?" I wondered.

"No, only normal licking," she said.

"Well," I said, trying hard not to laugh, "animal models for OCD have been described. What you read about is something called 'canine acral lick dermatitis.' These are dogs who compulsively lick their paws until they bleed, often getting serious infections. And as you said, studies of these dogs have suggested that SSRIs can actually stop the behavior."

"I hope our dogs never get OCD," she said, looking at George and appearing more anxious at the remote possibility of this problem than satisfied with my explanation.

"Don't worry," I tried to reassure her. "This is an extremely rare condition, so you should feel completely free to recycle that article!"

"But what if they do?" she said, her anxiety escalating even further at the idea of recycling something. "What if one of my dogs catches OCD one day, and I have to reread the article?"

"I can see Mother Superior hasn't completely taken care of the hoarder in you," George interrupted, chuckling.

I chuckled, too, and after a long pause, so did George's wife.

Later, watching George walk away from my office, his arm wrapped around his wife's waist, all I could think was how satisfying my cold pizza was going to be. With anticipation, I reached for the carefully wrapped wedge, slowly undoing the aluminum foil as I comfortably plopped myself in the oversized patient chair, turning it around so I could face the window. I propped my feet on the windowsill and prepared to take my first bite. But just as I was about to do so, an interesting scene unfolding in the parking lot outside my window caught my eye. I saw Dawn, all in black in observance of Good Friday, trying to catch up with George's wife, carrying what looked like a tall stack of magazines she had saved for her. George's wife gave her a big hug but declined the apparent gift, as suggested by Dawn energetically tossing the entire stack into the dumpster. The three then conversed briefly before George opened his trunk, and all joined forces to pull out a familiar-looking old table, each holding one of three remaining legs.

Pizza never tasted so good.

H$_2$O under the Bridge

As a psychiatrist, I am used to receiving referrals from internists and primary care providers, from other psychiatrists or specialists seeking a "second opinion," and of course, from concerned family members who sometimes have to force loved ones into my office for an evaluation against their will. But imagine my surprise at receiving a consultation request one morning from a worried . . . hairdresser!

"Dr. A., I'm so glad I caught you," a soft, earnest voice said. "This is Sebastian from Sebastian's Guild Salon in San Francisco."

"Do I know you?" I asked.

"No, we've never met before," Sebastian said, "but I understand you specialize in trichotillomania."

Sebastian's precise and deliberate pronunciation of the difficult word indicated perhaps a more than casual level of familiarity with the disease. "Have you been diagnosed with trichotillomania?" I asked.

"God, no!" he exclaimed, "unless you consider baldness a natural form of trichotillomania . . ."

"No, baldness is quite different," I said, appreciating the caller's attempt at levity.

Then, injecting a good dose of drama into every superlative, Sebastian added, "Well, if I still had my hair, the very last thing I would do is compulsively pull it out! I simply love and respect hair too much . . . This is not about me, Doctor, but about my dearest friend—who is also a top client of mine. She has the worst case of trichotillomania you have ever seen. I've worked with her for almost ten years now, but as creative as I am with hair—and I'm pretty good at what I do!—I've finally run out of tricks to cover up her bald spots. They're bigger than ever now, and I have less of her hair to work with, so I am officially giving up and asking for your intervention."

"Why doesn't she come in for a consultation?" I asked.

"She won't come in alone," Sebastian answered. "She needs me for moral support, she says, even though she might change her mind if she spoke to you. You seem very nice and, umm, quite friendly for a shrink. Forgive my prejudice, Doctor, but I've had some awful experiences with your profession in my day. This is not about me, so I won't go into how I was restrained against my will and given medications intramuscularly—*intramuscularly!*—or how I was court-ordered to get shock therapy—*shock therapy!* But, thankfully, all that is behind me now. H₂O under the bridge . . . So, going back to my friend Pat, I really do think you would find me quite helpful if I came in with her. I don't know if you know this, but hairdressers are their clients' confidants, and I can give you quite a bit of important information about Pat that she may have forgotten—or that she may not even know about herself!"

Although quite worried about what I was agreeing to, and about the considerable additional baggage Sebastian was sure to add to the mix, I could not create obstacles to Pat's first visit when she seemed to be in such great need of help. "If Pat is OK with your accompanying her, I am OK with it, too," I said. "Let's all meet and go from there."

"Sounds good," Sebastian said. Then, taking on an even more theatrical air, he added, "I do have one last question, Doctor. It's for my own personal peace of mind, really. Do you think I've been enabling Pat's behavior all these years by doing such a good job covering up her bald spots? I'm so very guilt-ridden by that thought! It just breaks my heart to think I may have been part of the problem instead of being part of the solution. To think that, for years, I jokingly called her Loulou, even giving her a parrot for Christmas one year, instead of pushing her into treatment, causes me intractable insomnia. Please, Doctor, tell me that I have not contributed to my best friend's devastating problem . . ."

Sebastian was referring to Loulou, the world's best example of trichotillomania across species, a parrot from a French novella by Flaubert with "his front blue, and his throat golden," who displayed a "tiresome mania" of compulsively plucking his own feathers. As delivered by Sebastian, however, this obscure literary reference came across as more show-offish than cultured. His penchant for high drama, combined with his feeling of victimization by psychiatry, made for an intriguing but potentially combustible personality mix that left me both very curious and very nervous. Despite reminding myself that I would not be his doctor, I was already concerned about what role Sebastian would play in his best friend's treatment.

"I believe you wanted to help Pat the best way you knew," I said, trying to reassure him. "It's not unusual for patients with trichotillomania to go for many years before seeking professional help, and most of them don't have talented hairdressers helping them out! I doubt that Pat would have come to see me much sooner if you had not been involved all these years, though I cannot say that with complete certainty. I'm glad, however, that you have now decided to help her get psychiatric care. It's absolutely the right thing to do."

⁜⁘⁜

Literature beat medicine to a description of what would eventually be called trichotillomania when Flaubert's novella *A Simple Heart*, featuring the parrot Loulou, came out in 1876. It was later, in 1889, that Flaubert's compatriot, Dr. François Henri Hallopeau, a French dermatologist, coined a new term, *trichotillomania*, by combining the Greek roots for hair (*thrix*), pulling out (*tillein*), and madness (*mania*). More than a century later, dermatologists still see people with trichotillomania more than psychiatrists do, despite the psychological basis for the disorder and the absence of any dermatological interventions that can stop the behavior. (Dermatologists can, however, be very helpful in treating the damage that results from trichotillomania, such as skin irritation and infection of hair follicles.)

Although the usual course of trichotillomania has been well described, much is still unknown about its causes and treatments. It is estimated to affect around 1 percent of the population, with women being more at risk, although women may also be more likely to be included in the statistics because of a greater willingness to seek treatment, whether from a psychiatrist or a dermatologist.

Diagnostic Criteria for Trichotillomania

A. Recurrent pulling out of one's hair, resulting in hair loss.

B. Increased tension immediately before pulling or when trying to resist the urge to pull.

C. Pleasure or relief while pulling and immediately following.

D. The pulling is not better explained by a skin condition or other medical or psychiatric illness.

E. The pulling causes significant distress or disability.

Source: Adapted from the *Diagnostic and Statistical Manual of Mental Disorders*, 4th ed. Washington, DC: American Psychiatric Press, 1994.

The DSM-IV criteria used to diagnose trichotillomania, summarized above, include mounting anxiety immediately before the hair-pulling and pleasure and relief during and immediately following it.

The overwhelming anxiety people feel before the behavior and the relief that comes with the behavior are shared by other *impulse control disorders* as well, including kleptomania, pathological gambling disorder, and compulsive sexuality (although the last is not formally included in the DSM-IV). In all these conditions, the pathological behavior varies, but a thrilling sensation is present, which distinguishes them from OCD, where the patient rarely derives any pleasure from the compulsion. So, whether it is the hair pulling in trichotillomania, the shoplifting in kleptomania, the betting in pathological gambling, or the repetitive cruising for sex in compulsive sexuality, these behaviors are experienced as pleasurable, although the patient is also guilt-ridden and tortured by them and is usually well aware of their negative consequences and the long-term damage they cause.

The pleasurable aspect of impulse control disorders can make them more difficult to treat than OCD, because patients are being asked to relinquish an action that, although problematic, is also enjoyable on some level. Another consequence is that patients miss these behaviors and the thrill that accompanies them when they cut back, and they may feel restless and irritable as a result. This withdrawal-like state has been likened to the physiological withdrawal from addictive substances like alcohol and is, in part, why impulse control disorders have also been referred to as behavioral *addictions*. In fact, Laurie, a forty-year-old nurse I treat for trichotillomania, describes the struggle to resist her pulling urges as "getting the shakes" and compares this state to what her husband, a recovering alcoholic, felt when he abruptly stopped drinking.

Another feature that distinguishes impulse control disorders from OCD is that the behaviors seen in impulse control disorders are often acted out without awareness, almost unconsciously. Laurie, for instance, would often tell me, "I didn't catch myself pulling until it was too late" or "By the time I realized I was doing it, I had a bald spot already." Similarly, patients with impulse control disorders like kleptomania, pathological gambling disorder, or compulsive sexuality can feel so disconnected from reality and so out of touch with the risks they are running that they can momentarily justify the stealing, betting, or promiscuous behavior, minimizing what is at stake. In contrast, patients with OCD are usually very conscious of their behaviors and often keep detailed mental or written lists of the compulsions performed and the time spent performing them.

Yet similarities with OCD do exist, leading some experts to refer to impulse control disorders as *obsessive-compulsive spectrum condi-*

tions. The spectrum concept has been championed by Dr. Eric Hollander, a psychiatrist and researcher at Mt. Sinai Medical Center in New York, who has detailed important parallels among these disorders. For instance, in both OCD and impulse control disorders, people experience bothersome, intrusive thoughts. In someone with OCD, the intrusive thought may be an irrational contamination fear after shaking hands with a stranger. In someone with trichotillomania, the intrusive thought may focus on how one particular hair feels different in the way it touches the forehead. Further, the intrusive thought in both OCD and impulse control disorders is usually associated with an irresistible behavior the person feels compelled to perform, such as hand-washing in OCD or hair-pulling in trichotillomania. This behavior, whether it involves ten minutes of hand-washing in OCD or pulling out a particular hair that feels different in trichotillomania, is often repetitive, stereotyped, and acted out in rigid patterns.

Sebastian entered my office first: a lean forty-something man with deep-set black eyes, wearing a tight-fitting black pinstriped suit, the stripes only a slightly lighter shade of black. A third shade of black, in the form of a partially unbuttoned silk dress shirt, completed the outfit. His glistening, totally bald scalp competed for attention with a shiny silver chain around his neck and heavy rings on his fingers.

Pat followed just behind. As I reflexively do when I am expecting a patient with trichotillomania, I focused on her hair first. My initial impression was that it looked artificially perfect. The immobile, meticulously arranged fringe in front and the impossibly symmetric outward flips on the sides clearly indicated that

Pat was wearing a wig. As she shook my hand, I could feel the sweat and tremor in hers.

"I'm glad Sebastian called to make this appointment," she said. "I know it's overdue."

"I'm glad he did, too," I said. "I understand from my brief phone conversation with Sebastian that you have been suffering from trichotillomania for a long time."

"She has," Sebastian interjected. "Where do you want me to start?"

"Maybe we can have Pat start," I suggested.

"He knows me so well," Pat said, "and it's embarrassing for me to talk about this."

"Trichotillomania is probably more common than you think," I said, "and you're in the right place now to do something about it. We can take a break later if this becomes too much for you, but can you tell me how this problem began and how bad it has been lately?"

A long, heavy silence followed, interrupted by Sebastian's muddled outbursts as he tried to control his urge to speak on behalf of his friend. He distracted himself by rotating his rings and moving his swivel chair in semicircles.

"It would be easier for me to just take my wig off," Pat finally said, turning toward Sebastian as if to invite his help. "What you will see is worth a thousand words."

Before I could object to what seemed like an extreme gesture happening too early in our meeting, Sebastian sprang up and positioned himself behind Pat's chair, the speed and energy of the jump causing his chair to complete a full turn on its axis. Then, deftly working his palms underneath Pat's artificial locks, he squeezed both index fingers between scalp and wig, slightly loosening the wig before dramatically and quickly lifting it. Pat closed her eyes, as if she was too ashamed to face me.

My eyes, too, briefly closed. I felt like I was somehow violating Pat without meaning to. Before I could establish any rapport with her, before I could offer any meaningful reassurance, an embarrassing problem that she had steadfastly kept from medical professionals for years was now abruptly revealed before the clinical gaze of a complete stranger. Something about the way it had happened felt violent, and for a sad moment, I wished I could roll back the less than five minutes of our meeting and have another chance at my first interview with Pat. But of course there can only be one first interview, and despite my regrets about the course of events, I had to make an assessment of the problem that was now being presented for my evaluation.

The natural light brown hair that Pat's wig had concealed appeared brittle and uneven. It was pulled up and collected in an anemic bun on the vertex of her head. Three one-inch bald spots on the sides were visible through the thin strands that snaked their way back from her forehead. These spots appeared red, indicating inflammation from repetitive damage to the scalp. In part to cover up the bald spots, in part to cover up the redness from inflammation, brown makeup the color of her hair had been applied to the bald areas, complicating the patchwork of color and texture.

"See? That is all the hair I have left to work with," Sebastian said, as he regretfully shook his head, sounding unusually subdued and hardly desensitized to the sight. He then released Pat's bun very gently by pulling out the single needle-thin clip holding it, taking the utmost care not to lose one more precious hair in the process. Pat's natural strands fell down, showing a variety of lengths resulting from recurrent bouts of plucking.

"I have these creams I use," Pat said, opening her eyes to locate in her purse two tubes of steroid-based lotion. "My dermatologist prescribed them for me."

"Do they help?" I asked.

"Not really," Sebastian quickly answered. "And neither do all the hypoallergenic products I've prescribed," he added, stressing the "I." "We have a basket in my salon that my helpers jokingly call 'Pat's basket.' It contains a complete line of fragrance-free, dye-free, and paraben-free pomades, shampoos, and conditioners. Very expensive designer products that only our Pat gets to use."

"And what are parabens?" I asked.

"You haven't heard of parabens?" Sebastian retorted, shocked at my ignorance of a seemingly very important toxin.

"It's a poison in the estrogen family," he explained. "It's been shown to cause breast cancer. It's usually found in underarm deodorants, but many commercial hair products also have it."

"I'm not familiar with the research on parabens," I said, "but I'm not surprised that all these measures have not helped Pat. They rarely do in trichotillomania, unfortunately."

"So should I stop using these creams then?" Pat asked, pointing to the tubes in her hands. "I'm not fond of using steroids on my scalp, anyway. I heard they can cause hair loss. Just what I need!"

"Low-strength steroid creams that you apply to the skin should not cause hair loss," I said, trying to reassure her. "Dermatological interventions like these can help with the inflammation and infection that pulling can cause, but they do not deal with the fundamental cause of the problem. They address the consequences of the pulling but not the pulling itself. That is why a psychiatric approach has a much better chance of success."

" 'A psychiatric approach?' I don't like the sound of that!" Pat said, looking at Sebastian as though to enlist his sympathy by reminding him of the scars the "psychiatric approach" seemed to have left him with.

"*I* do," was Sebastian's quick answer, delivered forcefully as he stroked the wig he had placed on his lap. "We've been in denial about this for much too long, Pat."

"How long, Pat?" I asked. "How long have you had this problem?"

Pat paused a bit as though still pondering the benefits of a psychiatric approach, then answered, "I guess it started when I was fourteen or so. Back then, I would just twirl my hair. Innocent enough, right? But then I somehow discovered the joy of pulling, and I haven't been able to stop since."

"The *joy* of pulling?" I repeated after her, intrigued by her choice of words.

"Yes, pulling, for me, actually feels good," Pat answered. "It calms my nerves."

"She's even used the word *orgasmic* once—jokingly, of course— to describe the sensation," Sebastian ventured, lowering his voice and looking away from his friend as he pronounced "orgasmic."

"Sebastian!" Pat yelled, reprimanding him for crossing a boundary she clearly did not want crossed.

"Sorry, sweetheart," Sebastian said, sounding genuinely apologetic as he reached over to squeeze Pat's hand. "We have to be completely honest with the doctor if he is to help us."

"It's an anxiety-relieving behavior, Pat," I explained, "so it doesn't surprise me that you experience it as pleasurable—most people with trichotillomania do. That is one reason trichotillomania can sometimes be challenging to treat. I will be asking you to stop a behavior that, at some level, you find soothing." Then, after a brief pause, I added, "But saying you find the behavior soothing is simplistic, of course. Even though the behavior itself feels good, you obviously don't like the consequences, and you don't like the fact that you have the disease. You wouldn't be here if you did."

"I can absolutely, unequivocally, and without reservations, tell you that I hate the fact that I have bald spots!" echoed Pat, nodding in agreement as she squeezed Sebastian's hand more tightly.

⁂

The largest study to look at characteristics of people with trichotillomania shows an average age of thirteen for the start of hair pulling. Most people with trichotillomania find special qualities in the hairs they pull, preferring coarse, curly, or thick hairs, or hairs that they feel touch their skin in an uncomfortable way. Further, most can identify high-risk situations that are more likely to trigger pulling, such as driving, talking on the phone, reading in bed, or watching television. Finally, the severity of the behavior often correlates with the person's overall level of stress.

Although many people with trichotillomania pull hair from their scalps, pulling also commonly targets the eyebrows and eyelashes, as well as facial and pubic hair. In fact, the natural tendency for the disorder is to migrate over time, so that a person who started pulling hair from one site may, for reasons that are unclear but do not include running out of hair in the first site, switch to pulling from another location.

The resulting bald spots cause great embarrassment and guilt for the victim, who will often go to great lengths to hide them.

Commonly used cover-up strategies include creative hair styling, wigs, excessive makeup, hats, bandanas, and false eyelashes and eyebrows. The disfigurement can lead to avoidance of social situations, dating, sexual relationships, activities like swimming and other sports, and even exposure to windy places.

For our second appointment, Pat arrived alone, wearing the same wig she wore to our first meeting but with a brace around her neck.

"What happened to your neck?" I asked.

"It's acting up again," she said. "My right arm is so numb and tingly I can't get anything done. It happens every so often, usually when my pulling is out of control."

"What's the association between pulling your hair and numbness and tingling in your arm?" I inquired.

"Well, there's this area at the upper left side of the back of my neck, right about here, that I enjoy pulling from for some reason," Pat explained, slipping her right index finger under the brace to demonstrate the location and grimacing with pain as she did. "The problem is that this part of my neck is not easy to reach with my right hand, which is the hand I use for pulling. Well, imagine spending two to three hours a day, your right arm wrapped behind your neck, and your neck bent forward, as you focus on finding more hairs to pull. Now imagine doing this for years . . . Talk about repetitive motion injury! I have a bulging disc in my spine as a result, and it's causing pain to radiate down my right arm. The brace is to immobilize my neck so I can avoid surgery."

"And does the brace help with the pain?" I asked.

"Yes, it does, as long as I wear it," Pat answered.

"Does it help in other ways, too?" I asked. "Does it reduce pulling as well by preventing access to your favorite pulling spot?"

"Well, yes," Pat answered, "but that's one reason I take it off when I should be wearing it. When the urge to pull is too strong to ignore, I simply take the brace off."

"Despite the pain?" I asked.

"Despite the pain."

"Despite the threat of neck surgery?"

"Despite the threat of neck surgery. Isn't that crazy?"

Several medical complications have been associated with trichotillomania. The most common are skin-related problems, including irritation, folliculitis (inflammation of the hair follicles), and infections at the pulling site. But pain syndromes can occur, too. The prolonged, unnatural postures patients assume while pulling can lead to neck, shoulder, or back pain, even carpal tunnel syndrome, compounding the problem by adding physical disability to psychic anxiety and cosmetic damage.

A particularly worrisome medical complication is *trichobezoar*, an emergency that results from a hairball blocking the stomach in people who swallow their hairs. About half the patients with trichotillomania have oral rituals associated with hair pulling, like licking or biting the hairs, or running them between their teeth in flossing-like movements. Fortunately, swallowing the hairs is far less common. For unclear reasons, teenage girls seem to be at a higher risk for developing this serious complication. Though I have never personally encountered a case of trichobezoar, I always ask my patients whether they swallow their hair, and I monitor young women especially closely for this problem.

⊞∷⊟∷⊞

Aside from the customary holiday party every December, it is uncommon for me to run into staff members in nonclinic settings, in part because I live an hour's drive from my practice, so it was surprising to see someone who looked like Dawn walk past me while I sat reading the paper in my local shopping center café one morning. Although it had to be Dawn, as suggested by her pregnancy, swift walk, and customary outfit—flower-patterned scrubs and white leather clogs—there was also something strikingly different about her. It did not take me long to realize that it was her hair: a big, glittery pouf with small white baby's breath flowers peeking through. Her hairdo looked like the meticulous, fussy work of a true artist, but her head appeared strangely detached from the rest of her body.

"Dawn, is that you?" I yelled from my seat on the patio outside the cafe.

"Dr. A.!" Dawn yelled back, sounding surprised. "What brings you here?"

"What brings *me* here?" I asked back. "What brings *you* here, Ms. I'll-only-go-to-San-Francisco-to-deliver-at-Saint-Luke's-Hospital? You don't look to me like you're in labor!"

"You're right," Dawn said as she crossed into the patio and pulled up a chair at my table. "I shouldn't talk bad about the big city so much. Maybe it's because we can't afford to live here that I say I hate it. It would be torture to love it and not be able to afford living in it . . . Anyway, I don't think anyone would deny that San Francisco has a lot to offer."

"Like excellent hairstylists, apparently," I said.

"Oh, you noticed my hair?" Dawn sounded elated as she proudly but gingerly patted her hair.

"Of course I noticed your hair," I answered. "How could I not? It looks very elegant. Very, umm, poufy . . . What's the occasion?"

"Do you think my Hector will notice?" she asked, perhaps believing that such a transformation could go unnoticed.

"He'd better notice!" I said. "So tell me, what's the occasion?"

"Well, we're coming up on our fifteenth anniversary," Dawn explained, "and we're going out for a nice dinner with the girls tomorrow to celebrate, and I had this free hair treatment and styling coupon from that guy who comes in to see you . . ."

"We have a hairdresser among our patients?" I interrupted.

"You know who I mean," Dawn said, almost breathless. "Sebastian, from the Beauty Guild Salon. He brings Pat in sometimes. Remember him now? What a caring, fun guy! Well, he and I struck up a conversation the first time he brought her in, and he told me all about how hair quality suffers during pregnancy, something about how estrogen interacts with testosterone—which women also have, apparently—by way of parabens, which are in the air we breathe and are highly toxic! Or is it the other way around? I honestly don't remember . . . Anyway, he took one look at my hair and offered me a free massage—a *hair* massage, that is—and said he would throw the styling in for free, too, and I said, 'Well, how generous of you,' and he said, 'Well, that's the least I can do for my Pat. Just take care of my Pat and put in a good word for her with the doctor,' and I said, jokingly of course, 'Well, Dr. A. takes good care of all his patients, but this can't hurt . . .' So here I am. The massage was great, but maybe he went a little overboard with the styling . . . That should be OK, though. It's our fifteenth anniversary, after all!"

"Dawn, I don't know how I feel about us accepting gifts from patients, let alone patients' friends," I said, knowing exactly how I felt about it—that it can only rarely be justified. "I'm not sure this is ethical, and it can end up indirectly influencing treatment in unfair ways."

"Well, how about doctors accepting gifts from pharmaceutical company reps pushing their drugs?" Dawn retorted. "How is that different? We watch these cheerleaders go in and out of the hospital all the time . . . And they shower docs with gifts— much more expensive ones than a hair massage, I might add. Don't tell me that that doesn't influence treatment in unfair ways, that it doesn't make a doctor more likely to prescribe their product. Now how is *that* ethical, and I should be made to feel guilty about getting a free hair massage for my poor pregnant scalp?"

Dawn was making an excellent point, of course, and one that any physician who has ever accepted a gift from a drug company rep would have difficulty countering. So, softening my tone, I said, "I'm glad you enjoyed your salon treatment, Dawn. It is well deserved. Your hair looks lovely, and I am sure Hector will appreciate it, too. Happy anniversary!"

Feeling proud of the case she had just made on behalf of deprived medical front desk personnel, Dawn took a big sip of the cappuccino I had ordered for her. Then, feeling even more energized, she said, "You want to go say hello to Sebastian? His salon is right around the corner."

"And do what?" I asked, annoyed at her bringing Sebastian up again when all I wanted was one of the city's best cappuccinos. "Update him on Pat's progress without her presence or consent? Now, that would be a clear breech of confidentiality. I really don't think so."

Dawn knew not to argue the point. She had also shifted her attention to a little girl sitting with her mother at a table near us. The girl was reaching over, trying to pull a flower from Dawn's hair. Instinctively, Dawn pulled away; then, feeling around the top of her pouf, she found a flower that protruded a bit. With a quick movement that left her new hairdo intact, she pulled out a six-inch baby's breath stem and lovingly planted it in the little girl's golden curls.

"Aren't girls adorable?" she said to the girl's mother. "I can't get enough of them, but we already have three, so we're really hoping for a boy this time."

Unlike OCD, little is known about the biological basis of trichotillomania or the centers of the brain implicated in the disorder. One intriguing hypothesis is that it may represent a disinhibition of, or loss of control over, some hardwired grooming behaviors. The similar behavior of compulsive feather picking has been described in several bird species, and its careful study could provide important clues about the biology of this disease.

However, even in other species, it is important to rule out physical causes for losing hair before a trichotillomania diagnosis is made. For instance, some parrots seen compulsively plucking their feathers may carry giardia, a protozoan infection that can cause severe itching in birds. Treating these birds' infection usually cures the plucking behavior. Similarly, other conditions that may lead to hair loss in humans must be ruled out before a diagnosis of trichotillomania is confirmed. For example, a reactivation of syphilis, which can happen several years after the initial infection, can cause patchy hair loss. Hence, individuals presenting with hair loss should be asked about their sexual history to determine risk for syphilis, and appropriate blood tests that can identify *treponema pallidum*, the organism that causes syphilis, should be ordered in high-risk patients. This is particularly important with the reemergence of syphilis as a public health threat, especially among gay men, as a result of the unfortunate relaxation of safe sex practices that has accompanied the new treatments for AIDS. Of historical interest, Dr. Hallopeau, the French dermatologist who coined the diagnostic term *trichotillomania*, was a syphilis expert.

Further, any injury to the skin that affects hair follicles can lead to hair loss resembling trichotillomania. This includes self-mutilation and radiation therapy in patients with cancer. Medical conditions, such as hypothyroidism or fungal infections of the skin like ringworm infection, often cause hair loss, too. In these cases, pharmacological treatment with thyroid hormone or antifungals is often sufficient to allow the hair to grow back.

Still, a small percentage of patients experience hair loss that is neither self-induced, as in trichotillomania, nor caused by any recognized injury to the hair follicle or any known medical condition. These patients are likely to have *alopecia areata*, a poorly understood disorder affecting about 2 percent of the population and thought to result from the body's autoimmune attack on its own hair follicles. More severe forms include *alopecia totalis*, where all scalp hair is lost, and *alopecia universalis*, where all body hair falls out.

"Tell me, Pat," I said at our next meeting, "these urges to pull that you describe: what makes them better, and what make them worse?"

"Well, they certainly get worse around stress," Pat replied, "especially dating stress. I'm an attractive—except for my hair—and successful mortgage broker, forty-two, still single, and with no prospects for intimacy as long as I have this problem. The thought of finding myself in an intimate situation that might expose my problem is enough to send me into a panicked frenzy."

"So the bald spots prevent you from dating because they're too embarrassing, and when you do find the courage to date, the stress around that leads you to pull even more," I recapped.

"Exactly," Pat concurred. "It's a vicious circle, and I'm caught in the center of it! I haven't gone out on more than two dates with the same guy for a very long time. The likelihood of some form of intimacy taking place on the third date if things go well is too scary to contemplate . . . What if he crosses the four-foot normal social distance and gets into my personal space? What if he approaches me in bright light for a kiss and spots the thick brown foundation covering parts of my scalp? What if he runs his fingers through my hair? What if? What if? What if?"

"That is really tragic, Pat," I said. "The idea that even with men you do like, you have to resist seeing them a third time and feel forced to end things prematurely . . ."

"Absolutely," Pat said. "I always sabotage things to turn the guy off and avoid seeing him again. Like this last guy Sebastian introduced me to, who turned out exactly as Sebastian had described: a handsome, gentle, successful realtor—a nice Jewish boy, really. And did I say handsome? Well, it came up on our second date that his sister had OCD and, as kids, she would spend three hours in the shower every day while he waited patiently for his turn, and as a result, he now won't allow any of his clients to buy a house with less than two bathrooms . . . Well, instead of empathizing with his childhood experience or using it as an invitation to open up about my own personal struggles with rituals, I went on to make fun of his sister's OCD in the most insensitive way imaginable! And I wouldn't shut up! Imagine, half-bald me making fun of his poor sister's showering rituals! Talk about the pot calling the kettle black! Well, needless to say, the third date didn't happen . . . And when Sebastian started asking what went wrong, the best I could come up with was, 'Well why don't *you* date him if he's so perfect?' I don't have to tell you that I haven't forgiven myself for this fiasco yet . . ."

"So you were intentionally pretending to be a mean person to turn off a guy you really liked so he would not want to ask you out on a third date," I summarized.

Pat nodded, her eyes welling up. This painful real-life example of the consequences of her illness brought Pat's tragedy home to me. Her tears drew me in. More than at any point in my meetings with her, I was able to get past wig and brace to appreciate the real hurt that lay much deeper than the outside manifestations of her illness, disturbing as those were.

I struggled to show Pat I was caring without losing control over my own reservoir of feelings. My theory has always been that you have to project resilience and empathy, almost simultaneously. Any "breakdown" on my part could be interpreted by Pat as a sign of weakness or inexperience and might lead her to doubt that I possessed the emotional backbone and resolve needed to address her problem. On the other hand, by closely identifying with Pat and openly and transparently sharing my feelings with her, perhaps to the point of tearing up in her presence, I might become more "human" in her eyes, thus enhancing our doctor-patient bond. But is this not what Sebastian and other people close to her attempted to do, without lasting success, and are patients not looking for something different from their doctors?

And what about my own mental health? Should I not be protective of that, too? Is there not a limit to how much I can identify with patients' problems before I, too, succumb to depression, negatively affecting my own life and severely impairing my ability to help others? Should I not be more like an oncologist, a cancer specialist who empathically delivers bad news all day but who does not bring these tragedies home and is able to sleep peacefully at night?

My internal debate was interrupted when Pat's growing discomfort with the subject of dating and this sad memory started manifesting itself in pulling urges that she seemed close to acting on right there in my office. I could see her reach under her brace with her right hand to that favorite spot in the left upper back part of her neck. I shook my head in an effort to dissuade her from pulling, a gesture I hoped she would interpret as "Don't do it." I wanted her, instead, to process with me the negative emotions our conversation was bringing up and to discuss other ways to dissipate them.

But before I could say anything, I heard Pat's voice come out, almost pleading. "Please . . . just one more," she whispered. Then, withdrawing her hand from underneath the cumbersome brace, Pat reached for a much more conveniently located hair sticking out from the side of her wig. With a deliberate, firm motion, as she held the wig in place with her other hand, Pat pulled one more hair—from her wig. I may be imaging this, but I think I saw Pat's tense facial features immediately relax.

⊞⋯⊞

No agreement exists among mental health professionals on the treatment of trichotillomania. In the absence of large clinical studies to provide clear guidelines, treatment usually starts by focusing on what has been called *habit reversal*. This strategy borrows from cognitive behavioral therapy and includes increasing awareness of the pulling behavior, enhancing motivation to reduce pulling, using a *competing response* to substitute for pulling, using relaxation techniques to decrease the urge to pull, and *changing the internal monologue* that justifies pulling.

It is very common for people with trichotillomania to comment that, by the time they "catch" themselves pulling, it is too late and too much damage has already occurred. Increasing self-awareness aims to bring pulling into consciousness. I usually start by identifying with my patient the situations that are likely to trigger pulling. For example, after tracking my patient Laurie's trichotillomania problem over two weeks using a daily pulling log that I asked her to keep, it became apparent that Laurie's worst pulling occurred while driving. With this information, I could tailor an intervention that targeted this high-risk situation. I asked Laurie to keep a pair of gloves in her car to wear whenever she drove. This seemed to reduce her pulling by taking the tactile pleasure out of it.

Competing responses are more socially acceptable, harmless behaviors the person can substitute for pulling. These are usually objects that provide some tactile stimulation, such as a stress ball the person can squeeze when feeling an urge to pull, a rubber band to pull on, or a makeup brush to stroke.

Motivation enhancement helps people with trichotillomania understand and remember why they want to stop pulling. With the therapist's help, the patient develops a list of reasons for stopping. For Laurie, the list initially included feeling more comfortable in social situations, feeling like she did not have to explain herself to anyone, setting a good example for her children, and finding healthier ways to release anxiety. Laurie posted the list on her bathroom mirror to serve as a daily reminder. I kept a copy, too, updating it as needed based on Laurie's progress in therapy.

Changing the internal monologue involves confronting assumptions about pulling that provide justification for continuing the behavior. For example, instead of "I've done so much damage, what difference does it make if I pull one more hair?" the patient is taught to shift her thinking to "Hair pulling is like self-mutilation, and I deserve better than this." Instead of "I'll only pull one hair and stop," the puller is taught to say, "I've never been able to stop at one hair, so I'm not going to test myself."

As with OCD, anxiety can trigger trichotillomania. Relaxation training can diffuse stress, thereby reducing pulling. Helpful self-relaxation techniques include deep, rhythmic breathing, visualization of a pleasant, soothing scene, and progressive muscle relaxation where the person is taught to tighten and then relax each muscle group in sequence from the toes to the scalp. Patients practice these tools in the therapy session and then apply what they've learned in the outside world to reduce pulling when they feel anxious.

Research studies on medications for treating trichotillomania are limited but do suggest that the SSRIs and clomipramine—all serotonin-based drugs well established for OCD—can be helpful. However, for most people, medications should be combined with therapy, as this is likely to give better results than medications alone.

❖❖❖

"Treating trichotillomania can be long and difficult," I warned Pat, "but trichotillomania is treatable, and you shouldn't let the effort and time it might take us to control the symptoms discourage you."

"I've never been in treatment before," Pat said, "and I'm as motivated as I can be to get better."

"You told me you were most likely to pull while sitting at your computer at work," I said. "Here, I want you to take this stress ball. Keep it on your desk at all times and try clenching it in your fist when you feel the urge to pull."

I handed Pat a squeeze ball that a drug company rep had given me. I believe he meant it for my personal use—a way for me to handle stress on the job, so I would subliminally associate the relief I got from squeezing the ball with the product he was marketing. It had *Paxil* emblazoned all over it in phosphorescent blue.

The bright colors caught Pat's eye, and she seemed momentarily amused. She gave the Paxil ball a good squeeze and seemed to approve of its consistency. "I feel better already," she joked. Shortly after that, though, her amused look morphed into circumspection. "But the problem is, most of the time I'm not even conscious of pulling," she worried. "How can I reach for my squeeze ball if I'm not aware that I'm pulling in the first place?"

"Excellent point," I replied. "That is why there is a parallel component to this therapy to make you conscious of the behavior itself. It involves having you collect the hairs you pull every day and put them in individual envelopes with the date and number of hairs written on the outside of each envelope. You then bring the sealed envelopes with you to our weekly meetings, and we use them as an objective way to track your progress."

Hearing this, Pat's circumspection changed into utter disbelief. And not without some irritation. "Did I hear that right?" she protested, sounding both incredulous and annoyed. "You're asking me to bring a week's worth of hair stuffed in envelopes to your office every week? Is this a joke? Did I forget to mention that sometimes I lick the hairs I pull? Do you still want me to collect them? I'm sorry, but this is a bit on the disgusting side, and I find it hard to believe that people actually do it! I'm afraid your treatment, Doctor, is too embarrassing for this patient."

"I agree that there is an embarrassing aspect to this, Pat," I said. "But some people do it—and with good results, I might add. One way to look at this is to say that we would be using the embarrassment factor to our therapeutic advantage, almost as a motivator. Here's how it works: the fact that you are saving and counting the hairs will make you more aware of the behavior, and the embarrassment of having to produce these hairs in my office every week will discourage you from pulling."

"I still can't believe this," Pat continued, already sounding a bit more resigned and a bit more accepting of the unconventional treatment recommendation. "Can't I just take a pill? Paxil, for instance? I already have their ball! It really would be a lot cleaner . . ."

"It would, for sure," I agreed. "But in my experience, behavioral therapy is at least as likely to help with trichotillomania as medications are. Plus, it is free of side effects!"

"Unless you consider embarrassment a side effect, that is," Pat quipped.

"I consider embarrassment in this case to be part of the intervention's mechanism of action." I said. "I look forward to seeing you in a week. Just make sure you seal those envelopes!"

One week later, I was interrupted by a page from Dawn in the middle of a noon talk I was giving to students. I called her right back.

"Pat, our trichotillomania patient, just stopped by," Dawn said. "She says she's sick with a cold—although she sounded perfectly fine to me! Anyway, she said she needed to rest and wouldn't be able to make it for her weekly appointment today. She did drop off some paperwork for you to review, though. She said it was important that I get it to your desk soon."

"Do you know what it's about?" I asked.

"I haven't a clue," Dawn answered, "but it looks very official. Seven nicely sealed envelopes, all dated and numbered, although the numbers don't seem to follow any sequence. Insurance company correspondence would be my best guess."

"I think I know what this is about," I said, feeling a bit guilty at having Dawn unknowingly handle a patient's hair—especially hair that might have been licked! At the same time, I really did not want to go into a detailed explanation of what Pat and I were up to. This was a hairy Pandora's box best left closed for now.

"Just save the mail in her chart until her next visit," I said.

"I can sort through them now if you want," Dawn replied. "Her insurance probably just wants more documentation before they'll authorize more visits. You know how I can sweet-talk insurance companies into almost anything . . ."

"I know your clout with insurance companies, Dawn," I said, "but no, really, this should wait until Pat's next appointment . . . Have you had your lunch break yet?"

⚎⋯⚎

A week after depositing her first batch of seven envelopes with Dawn, Pat arrived with Sebastian for another appointment. While Pat looked a bit brighter that day, Sebastian seemed preoccupied and less at ease than I remembered from our first meeting.

"The neon writing has rubbed off on my hands," Pat announced at the outset of the session. "I think I need a new squeeze ball!"

"That's a good sign!" I replied. "It means you've been taking full advantage of it. You've been doing the hair-collecting part of the treatment, too; I got your envelopes last week."

"And I have another week's worth for you here," Sebastian added, opening his black leather messenger bag to produce a stack of seven sealed envelopes. He looked numb and somehow mechanical as he handed over the envelopes, with none of the drama I had come to expect from him. Pat looked away. "It was either me coming with Pat today to hand-deliver these to you or Pat mailing them to your office," Sebastian added. "She has a very difficult time bringing the envelopes in, although she is religious about collecting the hairs!"

A quick glance at the numbers written on the envelopes revealed a slow decrease in the hairs pulled, from around 150 some two weeks earlier to about 100 now.

"It looks like you are doing a better job controlling your pulling," I commented.

"I'm more conscious of it," Pat explained, "and that translates into better self-control. Plus, I *really* don't want to have to bring them here, so when I pull now, it's when the urge is impossible to resist and the squeeze ball fails to make it go away."

"May I interject something here?" Sebastian broke in, looking more animated. "I mean, that is all fine and dandy, but it seems to me like we're missing the point. We're not addressing the *root* of the problem, if you will excuse the pun. I mean, what is *causing* this? Why is she pulling in the first place? Why does someone as normal as Pat self-mutilate like this? I can't see how squeezing a ball or collecting saliva-soaked hair can be a long-term solution . . . A band-aid maybe, but as long as the deeper issues troubling her are not addressed, it seems to me that the problem is likely to come back again."

"Well, what do *you* think, Pat?" I asked.

"I'm torn," Pat answered. "Part of me says, 'Whatever works, I'll take it,' but another part craves some kind of explanation, some kind of answer."

"I can understand your frustration, Pat," I said, "but—as is the case with so many conditions in psychiatry, and in medicine in general—we are far better at fixing the problem than at telling you exactly why you were the unlucky person who got it. Take diabetes, for example—"

"But this is *not* diabetes!" Sebastian interrupted, becoming louder and more irritated. "Can't you see? Deep inside, Pat-the-patient hates Pat-the-person, and this is her way of punishing herself. We need your expertise in reversing this, so she can start believing she deserves better. Unless she starts liking herself again, she will never stop this self-mutilation nonsense . . . When I brought Pat in here, I was hoping you would help us get there. I suppose I could have had her work in my salon, sweeping hairs off the floor and stuffing them in envelopes all day long. I guess that would have fixed the problem, too, but I chose to bring her here instead, hoping for more than that!"

"I could not agree with you more that Pat deserves better than to have to deal with this problem," I said, trying hard to hide my irritation at Sebastian's interference in the treatment Pat and I had agreed on, and which already seemed to be bearing fruit. I felt that a change in treatment approach could sabotage Pat's recovery, now in progress. I also wondered about the role his own history of unsatisfying psychiatric treatment might be playing. "I just do not believe that spending hours in expensive therapy to try to come up with a story that may or may not be true about *why* Pat pulls her hair will ensure that the behavior goes away," I added.

"Well, and I can't see how stuffing hair in envelopes guarantees anything either," Sebastian snapped back.

Feeling that continued confrontation was unlikely to lead anywhere and hoping to talk with Pat alone at the next visit, I suggested we postpone any decisions regarding the future course of therapy until our next meeting, when we would have more data on Pat's progress. Then, clearly addressing Pat, I said, "My recommendation is for you to continue with the hair-collecting and squeeze-ball tools until I see you back in my office in one week." I then discreetly slipped a brand new phosphorescent stress ball into her bag.

⊞⋯⊟⋯⊞

There was no sign one week later, however, of Pat-the-patient or Pat-the-person. Not the following week, either—not for two long months after our fateful meeting. Her envelopes, though, kept arriving reliably in the mail; I could count on finding one in my inbox every day, neatly addressed to "Dr. A.," with a stamp from a flower series in the upper right corner and a discreetly written number in the upper left one, where her name and address would have been. Dawn, increasingly pregnant and by now, I'm sure of it, quite aware of the envelopes' content, kept filing them in Pat's ever-expanding chart. "This is one bursting-at-the-seams ex-patient chart that I dare not send to medical records," she sarcastically told me over lunch one day, winking. "It might get us in trouble . . ."

"Pat is not exactly an ex-patient, Dawn," I corrected. "Not with a piece of mail arriving from her every day . . . In a strange and unique way, Pat remains a very active patient."

"In a *very* strange and unique way," Dawn quipped. Then, after a brief pause, she added, "I just can't understand why she hasn't responded to our calls. It's been almost two months already. Maybe I should stop by Sebastian's salon and check on her. I'm thinking of getting a perm before the baby comes anyway. I also miss talking to him—he cracks me up and makes me think."

"Absolutely not, Dawn!" I interrupted. "Perm or not, you are not to have a conversation with Sebastian about our patient. That would be a breach of confidentiality, and I cannot allow it."

"My, my, are we short and testy!" Dawn exclaimed. "Who's the pregnant one here, Dr. A., huh?"

Besides the obvious ethical concerns around patient privacy issues, one explanation for my irritability with Dawn was my defensiveness around the mention of Sebastian, who, in a sense, had been right to confront me, although he could have done it more tactfully and without the I-could-have-told-her-to-do-that-myself attitude. Like him, doctors—and perhaps especially psychiatrists—want to understand the *why* behind the symptom and feel some insecurity admitting their ignorance. After all, as doctors, we are not only called upon to fix a problem; we have to try to explain it, too. Only after a satisfactory explanation can patients avoid the triggers that brought on the symptom in the first place and thus feel confident in their recovery and the permanence of the fix.

This powerful drive to explain mental illness has given rise over the years to some fabulously simplistic and often ultimately wrong hypotheses for mental disorders—from the "schizophrenogenic mom" whose aloof and diffident nature somehow led her child to start hearing voices as a young adult to, more recently, the conceptualization of major depression as simply a disease of "too little serotonin" that is easily treated with medications that raise the levels of this neurotransmitter in the brain. Doctors should feel less threatened answering "I don't know" to questions that push the boundaries of medical knowledge, and patients should not necessarily interpret this "I don't know" to mean "I can't help you."

But even in the midst of my defensiveness around my inability to produce a satisfying cause-and-effect story to explain Pat's pulling, I could not help but notice that the discreetly written numbers in the upper left corner of Pat's daily envelope continued their steady decrease, from around 150 on the envelope at the bottom of the pile to less than 15 as the two-month anniversary of our last meeting approached.

Then, at exactly two months after our last encounter, Dawn paged me with her phone number followed by 9–1–1. I called her right back. "What's the emergency, Dawn?" I asked.

"Dr. A.! Pat is here!" she answered, out of breath. "She wanted to personally drop off an envelope with me, but I told her I wasn't comfortable playing the intermediary for her anymore, and she would have to give it to you in person this time. Should I schedule an appointment for her, or . . .

"I suppose I can squeeze her in right now," I interrupted, trying to downplay my excitement at seeing Pat again. "Have her come up," I said. "No! Dawn, wait! Is she alone?"

"Yes, she is. Don't worry!" Dawn reassured me. "I'll send her right up."

Barely two minutes later, Pat and I were sitting face-to-face in my office. She exuded an air of both refined elegance and serious business in her white pantsuit with oversized lapel, decorated with a large sunburst brooch whose shiny silver surface echoed the large metal hoop handles of her white leather purse.

It was a mark of undeniable progress that I was struck by other aspects of Pat's appearance before focusing on her hair. Pat was no longer presenting herself as someone who, because of deformity or extreme self-consciousness, was working hard to go unnoticed. That afternoon in my office, Pat *had* a physical presence, and a self-assured, attractive one at that! As to her hair, it was not lifeless or perfectly symmetric (as in fake), not overly luscious or flowing (as in exaggerated hair product advertisements), and not uneven, brittle, or combed-over (as in "trich hair"). It was pulled back in a neat-looking bun on the vertex of her head, with no random hairs sticking out from the bun or the sides, and no evidence of redness, bald spots, or makeup on the scalp underneath.

"You look very good, Pat!" I exclaimed. "But where have you been?!"

"I have something to give you," she said, avoiding my query into her extended absence.

"OK, but you did not answer my question," I insisted. "It's been two months!"

Before I could press her further, Pat slowly separated the large silver hoops of her bag, then quickly snapped it open to reveal a familiar-looking envelope.

"Please open it," she requested, handing me the envelope. "I'll explain—or try to explain—afterward."

My hesitation and confusion must have been visible as I assessed the envelope, which carried neither the customary flower series stamp nor the number of hairs on it. Just "Dr. A." in large script.

"Just open it," Pat insisted. "That's the last thing I will ask you to do for me."

So I did. I opened the white envelope labeled "Dr. A." and found it completely empty inside . . .

"I'm down to zero!" Pat said, flashing a big smile.

"That's great news, Pat!" I said, my surprise visible. "I'm proud of you."

"I do feel like I owe you an explanation, though," she said. "After our last meeting, I felt like . . ."

"You don't really *owe* me an explanation, Pat," I interrupted. "Feel free to explain yourself if you want, but you don't 'owe me an explanation.' I was just worried about you, and I'm thrilled to see that you are doing so much better now."

"I'm doing better for sure," Pat said. "In fact, I can't stay too long! I'm meeting my date in a half-hour."

"You're starting to date again! That's as good a sign as any that things have drastically improved. Is it the same nice Jewish boy you liked so much, by any chance?" I asked, excited that a promising, prematurely aborted relationship might get another chance. "He seemed to really like you, too, as I recall, but you sabotaged the whole thing out of embarrassment that he might find out."

"Who? God, no!" Pat said, letting out a loud laugh. "Didn't you hear? Well, there's no reason why you should have heard . . ."

"Didn't I hear what, Pat?" I asked, intrigued.

"Well, it turns out he was . . . Well, he and Sebastian are, umm, together . . ." Pat said hesitantly. "As like, dating each other," she added. "In fact, Sebastian perceived you as wanting me to pursue my relationship with Neil—that's the guy's name—which I think made him a little jealous. In retrospect, that explains some of his outright hostility toward you last time we all met. I'm very sorry about that, by the way. You didn't deserve it at all!"

"That's OK," I said. "H₂O under the bridge, as Sebastian would say. But I must tell you I'm very confused now. Wasn't Sebastian the one who introduced you to Neil in the first place?"

"He did, he did," Pat conceded, "but I'm now convinced that he was using me to test some hypothesis he had about the guy all along. Frankly, I'm confused, too. I could sense Neil *was* interested in me, but I also know he's seeing Sebastian now. Maybe he's bisexual or something . . . Anyway, it doesn't take a psychiatrist to guess that I'm a little mad at Sebastian right now. But it's nothing that he and I won't get over in time."

"Well, this is all very fascinating but also very sad, Pat," I said, wanting to give her an opportunity to process her feelings around what had happened. "I know how close you and Sebastian were, and I hope you can salvage your friendship."

But the nondoctor part of me was also simply curious, in a way that was perhaps inappropriate—more gossipy than clinically relevant to my patient. "Tell me more!" I said. "Do you think the two of them are a good match?"

Fortunately, however, Pat would not indulge me. "Well, I could go on and on analyzing this," she said, "but what purpose would it serve besides prolonging the same pointless drama? The fact is, I've moved on, and it's all H₂O under the bridge at this point . . . Plus, you don't want me to be late for my date, now, do you? Thanks for everything, Dr. A. Really, thank you."

With that, Pat stood up, gave me a hug, and disappeared into the labyrinthine hallway of our clinic, sounding a lot more confident in her step and a lot less anxious.

Yet my happiness at seeing Pat do so much better was somewhat spoiled by the sad suspicion that I would probably never see her again. I would never get the follow-up I was craving about all the new exciting possibilities in her life. I was also left with some cliff-hangers that I would never resolve to my satisfaction. But such is the lot of psychiatrists! Almost necessarily, we lose our patients right at the point when their lives are fullest and most interesting, right when we might want to be more, not less, involved. In wanting to watch our patients successfully navigate life, part of us—our ego—undoubtedly feels some pride for having helped them get there. Happily, however, Pat's problem was fixed, at least for now. Her life had taken off, and my role was officially over. I had to accept the fact that I would never see her again unless we were to meet at some awkward social function or she were to visit me in a disturbing Felliniesque dream.

But what to do with two months of hairy correspondence? Except for the final empty envelope, which I held tightly in my hands and then pinned to the wall in my office, I pushed the rest of the stack toward the edge of my desk, letting it drop off into the trash can. The thud of the falling pile as it hit the bottom caused a feeling in me that, however tinged by a sense of loss and separation, I can still best describe as satisfaction.

⁑⁑⁑

The morning after my final meeting with Pat, I came in to find an ecstatic message on my voicemail: "Dr. A.! This is Hector, Dawn's husband. Dawn delivered last night at Saint Luke's up in the city. I'm happy to report that we're the proud parents of a baby boy! We wanted to name him after a saint, so Dawn picked Sebastian, Sebastian Zuniga Ortiz. He's a big guy, too . . . Nine pounds and a full head of hair!"

A Greek Tragedy

"Did Jane Austen turn me on to kleptomania or did kleptomania turn me on to Jane Austen? It's a fascinating question to ponder." With these words, Hannah, my new forty-eight-year-old patient, a comparative literature professor and Jane Austen expert, tried to recall for me the origins of her urge to steal. "I was a senior in college writing my thesis on how Jane Austen transcended the boring details of her day-to-day life to write brilliant works of literature," she added. "I was looking in her biography for something surprising, maybe a little dark, that might have inspired her, but all I could find was story after story of Jane Austen as the dutiful sister tending her invalid brother or Jane Austen as the doting aunt—Jane Austen as the quintessential old maid, basically. And then, when I was about to give up on finding anything truly interesting, I came across court records about charges repeatedly brought against her aunt, Jane Leigh-Perrot, for multiple thefts. Well, my imagination ran with that! I started thinking how even the most serene and imperturbable of surfaces—like the social order she described so beautifully in her novels—can have undercurrents of sin and transgression running below their shallow waters. I imagined what Jane Austen might have written about her aunt the thief had she been able to publicly address this family secret. And given that she did not really write about it, I wondered how it might have indirectly informed her writing and whether the shame somehow found sublimation in beautiful prose . . .

"As I said, I don't recall which came first, and I certainly cannot blame my stealing on Jane Austen, but around the time I started researching the kind of lace Jane Leigh-Perrot was given to stealing, I, Hannah P. Wells, started stealing, too."

⊠⋯⊠

"Who the hell is Jane Austen?" asked Tenisha. I had just recounted the story of Jane Austen's aunt in an attempt to soothe her feelings of guilt and isolation, but it didn't seem to be having the desired effect. She had been court-ordered to see me in lieu of going to jail after giving powerful testimony in court that could serve as a definition of kleptomania, although Tenisha had never heard the term before. At our first meeting, she recounted for me her experience with stealing, as she had done with the judge who sent her to my clinic.

"Yes," she said, "we live in Section 8 housing, and, yes, I'm a single black mother with a boy who has sickle cell, and, yes, we live under a lot of stress. But the things I steal I don't even want! My last arrest was for taking a pacifier, for God's sake. A pacifier! Now you tell me—what need do I have for a pacifier when my boy is five? And why not buy it if I had to have it? We may live welfare check to welfare check, but I can always afford to buy a stupid pacifier or whatever other small things I usually steal! Listen, I grew up in the 'hood. I married a criminal. I've seen plenty of men in my day go in and out of jail for theft and other crimes, and I can tell you that my problem is different. I'm not saying I don't have one—God knows I do! What I *am* saying is that I'm not a thief, or I'm a different kind of thief, and that I don't belong in jail with my ex-husband and his friends."

"I agree with you, Tenisha," I said. "Your stealing is different, and you don't belong in jail. I know you didn't come here willingly, but that's because you didn't think that anyone else had this problem or that it could be treated. Well, this problem is a psychiatric disorder. It's more common than you think, and it has a name: kleptomania."

Since its introduction into the medical vocabulary in 1838, kleptomania has been the subject of intense controversy. The debate has focused on whether kleptomania constitutes a legitimate mental disorder to be diagnosed and treated by mental health professionals, or a form of willful deviance that is more akin to sociopathy and that is best addressed within the criminal justice system. Psychiatrists have generally supported the distinction between kleptomania and other forms of stealing, as evidenced by its inclusion in the DSM-IV, where kleptomania is defined as a repetitive failure to resist urges to steal things that are not needed for personal use or for their monetary value. The DSM-IV criteria for diagnosing kleptomania are listed on page 80.

Like other impulse control disorders, kleptomania is characterized by a strong urge to perform an act (stealing, in this case) that is pleasurable in the moment but causes significant long-term

Diagnostic Criteria for Kleptomania

A. Recurrent failure to resist impulses to steal objects that are not needed for personal use or for their monetary value.

B. Increased tension immediately before committing the theft.

C. Pleasure or relief at the time of committing the theft.

D. The stealing is not committed out of anger or vengeance.

E. The stealing is not better accounted for by sociopathy or other conditions.

Source: Adapted from the *Diagnostic and Statistical Manual of Mental Disorders*, 4th ed. Washington, DC: American Psychiatric Press, 1994.

guilt and remorse. More than any other impulse control disorder, the presence of guilt and remorse is crucial in establishing the kleptomania diagnosis, because that is what sets it apart from sociopathic stealing. Patients with kleptomania are tormented by guilt and find their urge to steal completely irrational—but irresistible. Sociopathic stealing, on the other hand, is usually not accompanied by guilt; it is heavily rationalized by the thief and always carried out for some desired gain. Examples of sociopathic stealing include stealing out of need, as when someone chooses to steal a head of lettuce for dinner; stealing for monetary value, like taking an expensive item to sell; stealing to show off, like when a teenager steals an electronic gadget to impress peers; stealing to support an expensive drug habit or a behavioral addiction like gambling; or stealing for purely sadistic reasons, as when the sole purpose is to torment another person.

The prevalence of kleptomania is unknown but has been estimated at 6 per 1,000 people, or about 1.2 million of the 200 million American adults. More women than men appear to suffer from the disorder, although a courtroom bias may help account for this discrepancy. Many thieves (and the lawyers representing them) try to use the kleptomania defense to soften the punishment and divert the case from the penal system to the psychiatric arena, and this argument is more likely to win over a jury and judge if the defendant is a woman. Hence, more women end up being evaluated by mental health professionals for kleptomania, possibly biasing the statistics.

Another bias is worth noting. The likelihood of the "kleptomania defense" succeeding increases with higher socioeconomic status, and the punishment seems inversely related.

⁂

Soon after receiving our first kleptomania referral, Dawn expressed a desire to make our offices "kleptomania-safe." That happened shortly before she went on maternity leave, and she saw it as a top priority that she needed to address before she could leave me "alone with some dangerous patients."

Dawn was finding her remarkable ability to empathize sorely challenged by this new crop of patients who were coming in with long criminal records and a history of jail time. In her opinion, this warranted a heightened level of vigilance and self-protection. Personally, I disliked the idea of clearing my work space of the little objects that gave it its character: mementos from my trips, tchotchkes from my years as a garage sale addict, and small gifts from former patients. Plus, the little data we have on kleptomania suggest that patients rarely steal from family members or friends, or even strangers. Rather, most thefts occur in large department stores (especially those with lax security!), where the victim is anonymous and it is easier for the kleptomaniac to justify the theft: "I only steal from rich corporations that can easily absorb the cost and never from the mom-and-pop corner store with the friendly owners who are barely making it!"

"I refuse to work in a sterile environment out of irrational fear!" I said to Dawn, rejecting her recommendation to remove pocket-size objects from my desk or alter anything about how we ran our clinic. "We have no reason to believe that these people, who are here to get help, will be anything but honest with us, and we should not assume that they will turn around and burglarize us! We just have to continue to be careful as we always are and to try to be understanding. Nobody else out there is."

"OK, just don't say I didn't warn you if something goes missing!" she said.

For patients with kleptomania, their behavior is always a "dirty little secret," but more so perhaps for Hannah, because of the outward perfection of the life she had built for herself. The tenured literature professorship, the "faculty ghetto" residence with a second home in the south of France, the successful entrepreneur husband, and the valedictorian son on his way to an East Coast Ivy League school—such visible signs of success abounded and pointed to an enviable life lived fully. How does one begin to insert kleptomania into such a fable-like landscape?

"Have you seen *Belle de jour?*" she asked in accentless French in one of our early meetings together.

"The movie with Catherine Deneuve? Absolutely!" I replied. "It's a French classic and one of my all-time favorites."

"Well, I know you're tempted to conceptualize me similarly," Hannah said, without any hint of self-doubt. "You know—the rich, adored wife, who grows a bit bored with her perfect existence so she decides to err on the wild side to spice things up—in Catherine Deneuve's character's case through submitting herself to violent sexual fantasies as a daytime prostitute and, in my case, through stealing and flirting with capture every time I do it."

"It sounds like *you* may be tempted to conceptualize your stealing that way," I said, reacting to Hannah's putting words into my mouth, especially when the words involved confident comparisons with daytime prostitutes. That said, there *was* some validity in this extreme analogy. "I would agree, however, that the thrill of getting away with something like theft can, for some people, add excitement and adventure to a life that is otherwise very comfortable but bland," I added. "But at what cost?"

"True," Hannah said. Then, after adjusting her position to an even more ladylike pose, she added, "I see a hole in this explanation of my symptoms, though. Unlike Catherine Deneuve's character, I don't consider my life bland—the Jane Austen biography I'm working on, for example, provides a good outlet for my passion, so that, professionally at least, I feel stimulated enough. But also in my family life and my marriage."

"I'm glad to hear that you feel fulfilled in all these spheres," I said. "But maybe there's another way to try to understand kleptomania in your case: not so much a rejection of boredom à la Catherine Deneuve in *Belle de Jour*, but rather of the societal rules that abound in bourgeois life. However, instead of openly and publicly challenging these rules—which would marginalize you in society and jeopardize the many comforts you appreciate in your life—perhaps you transform your rebellion into a secretive act of transgression that lets you express your anger but still gives the appearance of playing by the rules."

"What you're saying, then, is that I shift my anger," Hannah said. "I take the easy way out. I take my revenge on the department store instead."

"The problem, however, is that kleptomania is never an 'easy way out,'" I said. "In the mental calculus you do, it may seem like an *easier* way out, one that is less risky and less threatening to the social order, but that is true only if you don't get caught. But the overwhelming majority of kleptomaniacs do get caught—and think of the consequences when that happens!"

"So is my hatred for the fast-approaching tax day and the big check I have to write the reason why I stole a pack of cigarettes from the gas station yesterday?" Hannah asked, a hint of sarcasm in her voice. "Needless to say, I don't smoke. I even refuse to socialize with smokers!"

"I can't tell you with certainty why you stole a pack of cigarettes yesterday when you don't smoke and nobody you know does," I said, "but I do think it would be helpful to identify areas of frustration in your life, including rules that you abide by but don't believe in, and to try to address them head-on. However, while we explore those areas, it's also very important to implement basic antikleptomania measures to help you in the short term."

"I would appreciate that," Hannah said, lowering her voice and sounding more sad than sarcastic now. "I need some help in the *very* short term. I've been arrested twice already and have a court date coming up in three weeks. So far, I've been able to keep this from my husband because I've been able to avoid jail. My attorney is confident I can get off with only a weekend of community service this time but says I will likely go to jail if I get arrested a third time. Then my husband would find out, my comparative literature department would find out, and my life as I know it would be over. At the rate I'm going—three thefts a week—I see myself in jail before too long, maybe even before our next appointment. You can look for my mug shot on the front page sometime soon!"

Hannah's words were by now barely comprehensible, a combination of choking up on tears and the whispery voice of shame.

"Harm reduction is our first priority," I said, realizing the enormous stakes involved. "Three thefts a week is playing Russian roulette with your life. You absolutely must avoid all nonessential shopping until the urges abate. You may go to the store once a week to buy necessary things, but only if you are accompanied by someone: a girlfriend, your husband, your son, anyone. You don't have to tell them why you're bringing them along. And when you do go shopping, avoid baggy clothes or clothes with pockets and don't carry large bags—these make it easier for you to hide things. These are tools that are basic and self-evident, but they do work to some degree for many people. Follow them closely, and you *will* be here for your appointment next week."

Various psychotherapy approaches have been used to treat kleptomania but with inconsistent success. No evidence exists for the effectiveness of traditional psychoanalysis alone. However, understanding unconscious motivations for stealing can be helpful in some patients. This approach often employs tools borrowed from the Freudian or psychoanalytic school of therapy, but these tools are best accompanied by cognitive behavioral therapy, which encourages the patient to resist the impulse to steal while consciously creating obstacles to stealing. This approach also highlights the negative consequences of the behavior, and supplies patients with techniques for coping with the anxiety they will feel when resisting the urge to steal.

No guidelines exist for using medications to treat kleptomania, and doctors and patients wishing to consider medication treatment have only a handful of published reports to draw on. Still, such reports, along with well-designed drug studies in other impulse control disorders, can be a reasonable starting point in making medication decisions when psychotherapy alone is ineffective or not feasible.

※∴※

It didn't take Dawn asking me, "Dr. A., do you think you look forward a bit too much to your meetings with Tenisha?" for me to realize that I had a problem. Something about her appealed to me in a way that was beginning to raise the proverbial red flag in my mind—and apparently Dawn's as well. For starters, I had gotten into the habit of asking Dawn to schedule Tenisha's appointments at the very end of the day or right before my lunch break—two flexible time slots that allowed me to go over the thirty-minute session limit.

I greatly admired Tenisha for her remarkable resilience and tenacity. To her, kleptomania was another obstacle in a life rife with difficulties: racism, unemployment, incarceration, episodic homelessness, and single motherhood. And just as she had largely overcome the other problems, she was intent on overcoming this one, too, and I was intent on helping her in every way I could.

I told myself that Tenisha could barely afford to see me so I had to make sure she was getting her money's worth; she needed more education about psychiatric illness than my average patient and that took time; she needed more support than the average patient because of her limited social network; and so on. Yet, as much as I could justify to myself the extra time spent with her, I had to guard against countertransference, an old concept from psychoanalysis that is still very much alive and relevant, which cautions against letting the doctor's personal feelings toward the patient—good or bad—drive patient care. These feelings are often the result of unconscious processes that have more to do with the doctor than the patient. For instance, a doctor may take better care of a patient if her psychological or physical characteristics remind him of his beloved mother, or may ignore a patient's needs because something about him conjures up memories of a mean stepfather. Succumbing to these feelings and letting our fancy (i.e., positive countertransference) or dislike (i.e., negative countertransference) for a patient dictate treatment decisions can lead to the equivalent of nepotism and discrimination in health care.

Although counterintuitive, positive countertransference like what I was feeling toward Tenisha is as problematic as negative countertransference. Its symptoms include an overfriendliness and informality with the patient that can be harmful. If the doctor maintains a healthy distance from patients, they feel more comfortable divulging unacceptable thoughts and behaviors, such as kleptomania, or discussing, say, the sexual side effects of the prescribed antidepressant. There is a reason why patients do not share such information with their loved ones: it is often too embarrassing, and it puts them in a vulnerable position by creating an uneven playing field that may never correct itself. They also worry about burdening people they care about with their problems.

If the doctor comes across as too friendly or too casual, this manner can create a similar dynamic and impede sharing of crucial information.

It can also prevent doctors from asking sensitive questions in the first place, since these questions can feel too intrusive or socially inappropriate; if a patient reminds us of our mother, we may hesitate to ask a question we would never ask our mother. So, maintaining a respectful, formal distance offers safety and freedom for doctor and patient alike, and I was in danger of blurring this separation in my relationship with Tenisha.

And I was in danger of making the opposite mistake in my relationship with Hannah. The halo of perfection surrounding her persona had turned Hannah into an inaccessible superhuman in my eyes—a distant figure who was difficult to relate to. So much in her life was enviable that kleptomania pulled her back to earth—almost in a good way, I dared think—from the stratospheric heights where she functioned. Her direct or indirect comparisons between herself and Jane Austen or Catherine Deneuve did not help. I had trouble admitting it, but I did not look forward to my meetings with her nearly to the same degree as those with Tenisha. However, this was clearly my problem and not Hannah's, my "issue" and not Hannah's, and something I was morally and professionally bound to overcome so it would not affect my ability to treat her.

"Know thyself," applied to the doctor, is probably the best guard against negative and positive countertransference. Because of our training, which often includes psychotherapy, we are, as psychiatrists, generally better equipped than other specialists to recognize and address unconscious feelings that patients engender in us. For this reason, we should be held to an even higher standard when we allow personal preferences to interfere in the care we deliver to patients.

Before I could address my positive countertransference toward Tenisha, however, the criminal justice system intervened, forcing her to start adhering strictly to our appointment times.

"Here, Dr. A., I have something to show you," Tenisha said excitedly.

Then, slowly unzipping and taking off her knee-high black leather boot, she revealed a silver anklet superimposed on a black leather band wrapped around her lower left leg. She gently pushed the anklet down, exposing the leather band and causing the anklet's bell-like attachments to jingle a bit. "How do you like my new accessory?" she asked, pointing to the band.

"It goes well with the silver anklet," I said. "Nice contrast. But what is it, and why are you showing it to me?"

"I think it's cool, too," Tenisha answered, "but it's much more than the latest girlie accessory . . .

"Really? What is it, then?" I asked.

"My probation officer wants me to wear it," Tenisha answered, now sounding more serious. "I'm embarrassed to say that I violated my probation terms already. I failed to report to my probation officer last week."

"That's terrible. I'm sorry to hear that," I said. "What happened?"

"I was at the mall near my probation officer's building killing time until my meeting with him," Tenisha explained. "Bad idea, you're thinking, Tenisha killing time at the mall! Of course, but I thought to myself if there's one place on earth I wouldn't steal, it's from a store near the county probation department—I mean I could practically see his window from the store's cashiers' counter, I swear! Anyway, I thought I would be safe from my urges there, and I would be able to control them. Right? Wrong! I got possessed again. Something about these lacy pink baby booties I came across started calling my name: 'Tenisha, Tenisha, Tenisha. Aren't we cute? Do it! You know you want to do it. Do it! No one will ever find out. Do it!' Not voices or anything, more like my own thoughts going through my head. I will tell you this, Dr. A.: I battled the urge for a long time. I truly, honestly did. I thought of my boy and what would happen to him if I got caught again. I thought of the security guard I had seen at the bottom of the stairs. I thought of you and how you said this was an illness that could be treated. I fought these thoughts as hard as I could for a long time, walking in circles around the booties counter like a madwoman, but in the end, the thoughts were stronger. So, making sure there were no cameras filming and no one close by, I quickly tore the label off the booties' bag and stuffed them inside the empty travel coffee mug I was carrying. I then casually walked on to my probation officer's building across the street."

The degree of disbelief on Tenisha's face must have mirrored mine, and the "girlie" girl from a few moments earlier suddenly looked desperate and prematurely aged. "Is this sick or what?" she asked me, shaking her head. "I mean, what am I going to do next? Steal my probation officer's pen right from under his nose? I didn't get caught this time, and that's the good news, but by the time I was done circling around the booties counter and actually made it to his office, I was a full hour late, and he was gone for the day. The following morning, he shows up with two deputies at my door and gets me fitted with this monitoring device, and now I have to wear this *and* see you once a week for the rest of my probation time—that's sixty more days!—or go to jail. Also, except for coming here once a week—I have ninety minutes to do it, including travel time—and taking my son to school, I'm under house arrest. I also have to report back to court in four weeks to answer for the probation violation."

"I'm really sorry to hear that, Tenisha," I said. "It seems you fought really hard to resist the temptation to steal, and I want to give you credit for that and encourage you to continue trying to resist. One way to look at what happened is that it should keep you out of stores until our treatment can start working and the urges decrease. On the other hand, it *is* a point against you, and if you are ever arrested again—"

"I know," Tenisha interrupted. "If I'm arrested again, it's straight to jail, maybe even prison. This is California, 'three-strikes-and-you're-out' country!"

"We should maximize your chances of beating this, Tenisha," I said. "A lot of therapy for kleptomania is about helping patients avoid stores and making it more difficult for them to steal. Although I wouldn't have chosen it for you, the monitoring device will help by keeping you away from stores. But a small number of reports have shown that medications used for other compulsive conditions also decrease the urge to steal in some people with kleptomania. For that reason, I suggest starting Lexapro at the lowest dose, and seeing how you do on it. We have very little to lose . . . Ideally, if it works, you should see the urges to steal become less frequent and easier to resist."

Tenisha looked skeptical. "I have to be completely honest with you, Dr. A.," she said. "I have big doubts about medications in general, and especially for this. But I also know my son's life is at stake here, and I'll do anything for him."

"Give it your best shot, Tenisha," I said, handing her the prescription.

"I will. I can promise you that," Tenisha said earnestly. "Can I get going now?"

"I know we can't dilly-dally now that you're under house arrest," I said, "but you told me they gave you ninety minutes total to see me, including travel time, which means we still have fifteen minutes to go! That is enough to cover some therapy tools still."

"I know, I know," Tenisha said, "but I thought I'd stop by the Goodwill store on the way home . . . Those baby booties I stole are burning a hole in my conscience, and I think I'll feel better if I donate them to somebody who may actually have some use for them."

Besides providing clinical care for patients like Hannah and Tenisha, academic institutions like Stanford are also teaching and research centers, training the next generation of doctors and conducting studies that improve our understanding of diseases in a way that can lead to better treatment options. Our Obsessive Compulsive Research Program at Stanford is headed by Dr. Lorrin "Larry" Koran, a man I am proud to call my mentor. Everyone in the field knows Dr. Koran as a revered authority on OCD, but few besides his students, his patients, and those of us who work closely with him get to see his many other qualities, like his kindness and dedication and how seriously he takes his roles as doctor and teacher.

Nona Gamel, our research coordinator, is another indispensable member of our group. A former social worker and romance novelist, Nona combines superlative clinical acumen with a creative, innovative side—a winning combination for a researcher and a great asset to our group. I am fortunate to have her as a colleague and friend.

For Nona, Larry, and me, of all the studies we have done together, the kleptomania survey still generates the most passion. I think we are all more or less resolved not to do another kleptomania study. (The reasons for this, including the heart-wrenching, desperate consequences of kleptomania we witnessed, the frequent no-shows by many subjects who questioned our motives, the court appearances we were asked to make, and the sociopaths masquerading as kleptomaniacs with whom we had to interact, would make a great subject for another book!) However, I also think that we all feel somehow stronger because of this study, as though we can weather any research-related obstacle we may encounter in the future after having successfully interviewed probably more kleptomaniacs than anybody else. So what did we learn?

Using radio and newspaper ads, as well as referrals from the court system and from other doctors, our group recruited forty individuals meeting DSM-IV diagnostic criteria for kleptomania. Subjects were carefully screened to exclude those who did not fit the kleptomania model before a comprehensive psychiatric interview was done.

Most subjects in our study were women. On average, they began stealing at seventeen, although a third of them reported stealing even before age eleven. After the first appearance of the behavior, most subjects had a continuous course with only brief kleptomania-free periods. Our study also highlighted the serious legal consequences of this disorder: over 75 percent of subjects had been arrested for shoplifting.

Only 5 percent of subjects in our study had received medications specifically for kleptomania, although nearly half had received pharmacological treatment for coexisting psychiatric conditions. This may reflect patients' confidentiality concerns about disclosing to their doctor a problem that is illegal, or it may reflect the reluctance of medical professionals to accept kleptomania as a treatable illness.

⬚⬚⬚

With Dawn now on maternity leave, I was left to my own haphazard scheduling, leading to appointment mix-ups, increased conflict with insurance companies, lengthy delays in processing new patients, and other logistical mistakes that Dawn would have never allowed. One such mistake occurred early one Monday morning, when I walked into my waiting room to find two patients waiting to see me for their eight o'clock appointment. I had double-booked, and the two victims were the two kleptomaniacs in my practice, Hannah and Tenisha.

The striking juxtaposition of the two women sitting on opposite ends of a couch was enough to jolt me out of any residual morning lethargy and into a state of hyperalertness.

"Good morning, Dr. A.," Hannah and Tenisha said, almost in unison, as one gently set aside a copy of the *Economist* magazine and the other dropped her issue of *Cosmopolitan*.

"Good morning, ladies," I answered, stupefied, as I took in the scene. There was Hannah, in her prim and proper beige pantsuit, her hair pulled back to reveal a face free of both makeup and emotion. Her leather briefcase sat on the floor nearby. On the opposite end was Tenisha, wearing a short black imitation leather skirt, with matching knee-high black boots covering most of the rest of her legs, and smelling of tobacco and cheap perfume mixed together. A furry black and white backpack with a flap lid in the form of a polar bear head with claws sat next to her on the couch. Tenisha's broad smile on seeing me was almost too much emotion to take in so early in the morning.

Despite looking worlds apart, Hannah and Tenisha, probably for the first time in their contrasting lives, were true equals that Monday morning, united on the same couch by one diagnosis and one doctor's hapless state in the absence of his able office clerk. What followed was a delicate acrobatic act to explain my mistake to the two women without divulging even first names and without making it obvious to either one that her neighbor on the couch was a psychiatric patient, too, let alone one who suffered from kleptomania. Knowing Tenisha was under strict house arrest, I suggested that I meet with "the lady in black" first, to which Hannah graciously agreed.

⊞∷⊞

Tenisha started out joking about finding ways to outsmart the satellite system monitoring her every move. "It's crazy-making," she complained. "The other day I went after my son when he ran over to the neighbor's to play, but as soon as I crossed the edge of our lawn, the satellite immediately called my probation officer, who then called me. He was so quick, you'd think I was the only person in the whole wide county he was monitoring! You'd think they had a whole satellite up in the sky tracking down poor Tenisha! You know, Doc, how some people will pay a lot of money to get a star named after them? Well, I have a satellite named after me, and it didn't cost me nothing! Anyway, good thing I was able to run back into the house and answer him. And while I was on the phone with him, I asked if he would allow me to have a longer leash, so I could at least go buy food for my son, instead of depending on my neighbor. He refused. 'Not even to the grocery store?' I asked him. '*Especially* not to the grocery store,' he answered."

I could only laugh with Tenisha and appreciate her perspective on the situation and her ability to fish for humor in the darkest of swamps. To her, life was a tragicomedy: laugh at it while you try fixing it, and if the fix proves elusive, at least you will have had the laughs! For a split second, I found myself tempted to offer to get her food for her, or to give her whatever I had in my clinic fridge. But realizing that this would likely be succumbing to countertransference, I opted to turn the conversation back to purely clinical matters.

"You've been on the Lexapro for two weeks now," I said. "Any side effects? Any good effects?"

"No side effects, and I've been taking it every day, I swear!" Tenisha answered. "I don't know if I'm reading too much into this, but I must say I haven't thought about stealing for about a week. It's probably because the opportunity hasn't come up, being under house arrest and all."

"Well, that is encouraging, Tenisha," I said, "although it probably is a bit too early to see the full medication effect. Continue taking it every day like you have been. Also, tempted though you may be to outsmart the satellite system, please try to resist doing so! Nothing good can come from it."

"Don't worry, I won't," Tenisha reassured me.

"One more thing," I said. "Remind me of when your court hearing is."

"In two weeks," Tenisha answered.

"Can I talk to your attorney?" I suggested. "Sometimes we can help by writing a letter that your attorney submits to the judge explaining what kleptomania is and how committed the patient is to treatment. No guarantees, of course, but it can't hurt."

"I don't have an attorney," Tenisha answered, in a matter-of-fact tone, as though she had grown accustomed to a legal system that did not ensure adequate representation for folks like her. "I can't afford one. It'll probably be some last-minute county-appointed guy with an expired license like last time."

"I cannot help find you an attorney, unfortunately, but I am going to write a letter on your behalf that I want you to present to the judge," I said. "I really hope it makes a difference."

There are many costs to kleptomania, not the least of which is the further burdening of our already overstretched criminal justice system. Approximately two million Americans are charged with shoplifting annually. If kleptomania accounts for 5 percent of these, this translates into 100,000 arrests, mostly on misdemeanor charges, although, based on the value of the stolen item and the person's criminal record, a felony charge may be considered. In the twenty or so states that have implemented laws similar to California's 1994 "Three Strikes and You're Out," this could mean longer—possibly lifetime—incarceration periods for kleptomania-motivated thefts.

Another way kleptomania affects the average citizen is through the inflated price of goods. Although only a small subset of the overall shoplifting problem is directly attributable to kleptomania, this is still a $500 million problem, based on total shoplifting estimates of $10 billion annually. Someone has to pay the price, and we all do. High as it is, though, this figure still underestimates the problem because many businesses do not report thefts.

❏⋯❏

"You know, Dr. A.," Hannah said, "these behavioral therapy interventions, as simple as they are, actually seem to be working! I've been ordering my groceries mostly online. I've been bringing my son with me for most of my other shopping needs. Of course, like most guys, he hates it, but he will come along when I remind him that he is about to leave for college and that his mother wants to spend as much time as possible with her only child before he does."

Then, after pausing to wipe a guilty look off her face, Hannah continued, "I couldn't bring my son along yesterday, though, because his birthday is coming up next week and I had to buy him a birthday present. So, as you recommended, I wore tight clothes with no pockets and didn't bring any bags with me. I carried my credit card in the palm of my hand. I also picked a local store that I know from previous experience has very tight security. I found an elegant watch for my son, which I paid for, but I was also tempted to steal an adorable Victorian jewelry box I saw. However, realizing that I had nowhere to hide it and that I was probably being filmed from at least two directions, I decided to hold back."

Hannah feared that her description of how she resisted stealing might have made it sound too easy, so she sought to assure me that it wasn't. "In no way do I want to imply that I had an easy time walking away from that jewelry box," she said. "I could still almost *physically* feel its smooth red velvety interior torturing my fingers as I walked out the door. It is just that the risk of getting caught was so undeniable in this case that I had no option but to leave the store empty-handed. Well, sort of empty-handed—I did have my son's watch, which I had paid for."

"The risk of getting caught was obvious because you had purposely set it up to be so," I said, "and this is in part the purpose of behavioral therapy. You try to create a deterrent to stealing by making it so complicated that you can no longer assume that you can get away with it. Congratulations on your success!"

"So," I continued, "with these interventions in place, can you tell me how much stealing you did this past week?"

"For the first time in a while, I haven't stolen at all this week," Hannah answered, "although I suspect that my approaching court date may have something to do with it as well."

"It's probably both," I said. "By the way, your lawyer called me about your court date and asked if I would write a supportive letter to the judge about your condition. With your consent, I'm happy to provide him with such a letter."

"You have my consent," Hannah said.

"He also seemed very confident that you would get off with only limited community service this time, just like last time. He seemed very experienced in these types of cases, and that should reassure you," I said. "It's a definite advantage."

<hr />

The timing of my discovery could not have been worse. As I sat in my office one afternoon, lazily waiting for inspiration to compose a strong letter to the judges who would decide the fate of my two kleptomania patients, I noticed that a turquoise-encrusted seashell ashtray I had bought on a trip to the Greek island of Santorini was missing from the table where it had sat for years, between the two swivel chairs where patients in my office usually sit. For a long time, I had used my Greek memento as a bright window to the Mediterranean on particularly gloomy days and, secondarily, as a business card holder. It had given countless patients the opportunity to break the ice by inquiring about its origins or its bright colors before delving into difficult emotional territory at the beginning of a session. It had also given them something to caress, feel, and play with, in lieu of biting their fingernails, wringing their hands, shaking, or otherwise manifesting anxiety or boredom. But once it had served its purpose, these patients invariably safely returned my prized Greek souvenir to its location, neatly restacking my business cards in it. Until, that is, somebody walked off with it.

How long my ashtray had been missing I could not tell, but I doubted that the after-hours cleaning staff had taken it. Even though they were the only ones to have access to the office in our absence, we had had the same stable crew for a long time, and I trusted them completely. It was also unlikely to be a nonpatient: I rarely held meetings in my office, preferring our conference room or the cafeteria for that. This left me with the uncomfortable suspicion that a patient must have taken it. As it turned out, there had been only two recent additions to my caseload, and both were kleptomaniacs!

So was it Hannah or Tenisha? I asked myself. My instinct was to blame Hannah immediately. At one of our earlier meetings, she had mentioned stealing a pack of cigarettes from a gas station (to take revenge for tax day, she joked!) even though she didn't smoke, so it seemed logical that she would steal an ashtray next! Although Hannah had stopped carrying a purse or wearing pocketed clothes to stores, she still carried her large briefcase and wore regular clothing to her appointments with me. And her son certainly didn't come along to keep her from doing it! In my mind, strong suspicion surrounded Hannah, and her attorney still had the boldness to request a letter from me asking the judge to mitigate her punishment!

But was I not being overprotective of Tenisha and unfair toward Hannah? Was I giving in to my countertransference once again—positive toward Tenisha and negative toward Hannah? After all, Tenisha had stolen from under her probation officer's nose, so why would I expect her to show more restraint in her shrink's office? Plus, a faint tobacco smell often trailed behind her, indicating that she was a smoker. How could I ignore all that?

I tried not to remember them, but Dawn's words before she left were ringing loudly in my ears: "Just don't say I didn't warn you if something goes missing!" I felt like calling her to commiserate but feared a self-satisfied "I told you so." Instead, I considered that it had been ten months since my last vacation and much, much longer since I had visited Greece, and decided to use this opportunity to plan a trip back.

But before I could rework my schedule to make room for an impromptu Mediterranean excursion, I had to finish the two letters I had promised to write on behalf of my two kleptomania patients on trial for shoplifting, regardless of how I felt about them at the time—which was more like an irate victim of their pathological behavior myself. It was no easy task by any means, but I finally found it in my heart to write what I thought was a forceful letter in support of the two women. The same letter, with the appropriate name, went out on official letterhead to each judge.

Dear Judge Reynolds/Byron:

I am writing to you on behalf of my patient, Ms. Tenisha L. Scott/Ms. Hannah P. Wells, who has been in psychiatric treatment in my practice for three months. I understand you will be presiding over a court hearing that will decide her punishment following a second shoplifting-related arrest, and I thought you might find my input to be of some value.

As you know, shoplifting is a serious crime that deserves appropriate retribution for the havoc it creates and the innocent victims it leaves behind. However, for a subset of shoplifters (those with kleptomania), the victims include the shoplifter. It is my clinical assessment that Ms. Scott's/Ms. Wells's shoplifting is consistent with kleptomania, insofar as it does not seem motivated by the classic factors that drive sociopathic stealing: monetary gain, drug use, the need to show off, the desire to inflict pain, etc. Rather, Ms. Scott's/Ms. Wells's shoplifting stems from an anxiety-ridden drive to steal items that are of limited or no use and that are easily affordable, and it is accompanied by tremendous guilt and remorse.

At its core, kleptomania shares many features with other impulse control disorders or behavioral addictions that we routinely treat in our practice and, like them, stands a reasonable chance of responding to psychotherapeutic or pharmacological interventions. For that reason, I feel that it would be better addressed in the psychiatric rather than the criminal justice arena.

Since the beginning of our work together, Ms. Scott/Ms. Wells has shown a genuine commitment to getting better and has been exemplary in adhering to appointment times and treatment recommendations. It is my hope that you will be able to take her clinical condition into consideration as you deliberate her fate, and that she will be given a chance to continue the psychiatric treatment that she needs and deserves.

I thank you for your consideration and, with Ms. Scott's/Ms. Wells's permission, stand ready to try to answer any questions you may have about kleptomania or my work with Ms. Scott/Ms. Wells.

Best regards,
Elias Aboujaoude, M.D.

"I'm so relieved," Hannah said, letting out a deep sigh, as she let herself fall into the oversized swivel chair in my office. "The judge took one look at your letter, said I didn't look like a shoplifter, and asked me what my 'strengths' were so he could tailor my community restitution! I thought to myself, gosh, what a nice man! I told him I was working on a Jane Austen biography, so he suggested a weekend of helping out at a halfway house for delinquent minority women. The idea is that I would use my language skills to help with disability paperwork, job applications, mock interviews, and so forth. He also encouraged me to continue my treatment with you."

"That's great news, Hannah," I said. "I'm relieved for you and glad that my letter seems to have helped. It will be important, though, not to assume that the threat of ending up back in court or even in jail is protection from ever stealing again. You should continue actively using the tools we talked about in a deliberate, conscious way."

"I will, and will continue to work with you for as long as you think is appropriate," Hannah answered.

"That is very encouraging to hear," I said. "Let's continue meeting weekly for now. I would like you to start a daily log of any kleptomania urges you feel, noting whether they were associated with any particular triggers, and how you dealt with these urges without, hopefully, acting on them."

"That sounds good," Hannah agreed. "Even though I haven't started the log yet, I can tell you I haven't shoplifted since our last meeting," Hannah answered.

"Very good," I said. Then, looking for clues about my missing ashtray, I asked, "You know, we focus on 'shoplifting' but people with kleptomania can engage in other forms of stealing too. So how about stealing from other sources besides stores? As in stealing from regular people, public buildings, professionals you may be interacting with? That also counts as stealing!"

" 'Stealing from other sources besides stores'? Oh, no!" Hannah answered, sounding outraged at such a possibility. "That has never been a problem for me, fortunately. Can people really do that and still call themselves kleptomaniacs? It wreaks of sociopathy to me!"

I was already feeling some guilt about my indirect inquiry into whether Hannah stole my ashtray. Somehow, it felt self-serving and unfair despite the 50 percent chance that she had taken it. However, I was made to feel even guiltier at the end of our session, when Hannah opened her briefcase to reveal an elegantly wrapped rectangular box—a thank-you gift for the letter I had written to the judge. I thanked her and, after she left, opened the present to find a highly ornate new collector's edition of Jane Austen's *Pride and Prejudice*. Its first page was signed, "With gratitude, pride, and no prejudice, HPW."

━━━

I should have known it, of course. Greece was too ambitious a vacation for my schedule to handle, so I had to settle on a warm destination that was more accessible—Las Vegas! I had brought Hannah's novel along for the plane ride and for those lazy resort afternoons by the pool but ended up not touching it, justifying this by telling myself that it was too nice to take out of its leather casing, and it wasn't exactly vacation reading anyway. Not to mention the weather, which turned out to be unseasonably cold for lounging poolside.

Given that I did not particularly enjoy gambling and did not want to spend my time on the casino floor, this left shopping as my main pastime. However, while Las Vegas's myriad stores did not carry Greek seashell-encrusted ashtrays, or even made-in-China imitations thereof, I did find a phosphorescent mint dispenser shaped like a slot machine that I bought—a relevant memento, I thought, for a clinic that treated behavioral addictions, including pathological gambling.

Back in the office, before I could spend time making room on my cramped shelves for my new purchase, I had to empty my inbox. Two items stood out and seemed to immediately recalibrate my mindset back to its pre–Las Vegas state: a letter from Tenisha and a box from Dawn with a note attached.

Dear Dr. A.,

I apologize for writing on such paper and with a pencil, but it's all I have here in jail. Obviously, the hearing didn't go well. The judge didn't even read your letter. He took one look at me and started lecturing me about shoplifting and how terrible it is and how terrible I am for burdening the economy and our legal system . . . Yes, Tenisha is now the straw that will break the back of our economy and legal system!

I'm very worried how all this will affect my son. He had to be moved to Atlanta to be with his grandmother. Poor baby! Give him a couple of years and he'll be in your office himself but, I pray to God, with a better disease than his mother!

I must tell you before I forget, though, that your medication seemed to be working! I was having less urges for sure, but they said the jail pharmacy didn't carry it, so I've had to stop. I know it's a very crazy thing to say, being in jail and all, but I can really feel those damn urges coming back!

Sincerely yours,

Tenisha L. Scott

Dear Dr. A.,

Did you realize this went missing? I was hoping, with all the stuff you've brought back from your trips (you sure travel a lot!), that you wouldn't. Anyway, I knocked it over trying to replenish your business cards on my last day before going on leave. Not to worry, though. Hector was able to find an antique guy who did a beautiful job restoring it! You can still see a hairline fracture between the shells, but only if you look really, really close.

Sorry for any inconvenience and see you in about two weeks. I will try to pop in with Sebastian for a short visit before then. I know you're dying to meet him!

Best,

Dawn

With Any Luck

I met Mr. and Mrs. Kuong at a moment of transition: before a move they were planning from California to Utah and after they had moved to California from Las Vegas. A striking Chinese American woman with porcelain-white skin and wearing a black pantsuit with a red kerchief tied around her neck, Mrs. Kuong at first glance looked more like the daughter than the extraordinarily well-preserved wife of the shuffling, graying man hiding behind her as she walked into my office, led by Dawn.

"It is important that I start at the beginning, from point zero," Mrs. Kuong said, not waiting for me to ask the opening question or even to address her husband, whom Dawn had introduced to me as the patient. "As I sit here, I can't say that I am too optimistic," Mrs. Kuong added. "We may be too far gone for you to be able to help us, and our only realistic option may be to move yet again. But if we can't be helped, maybe we can be of help. Maybe we can serve, through you, as a lesson to other patients at less advanced stages. I like to think that some good can come from our story."

After this foreboding introduction, Mrs. Kuong readjusted her position in the chair, as if preparing for a long, almost physically painful narration of their tale.

"So let me start from the beginning, please," she repeated. "We got married young but not by those days' standards. I was twenty and studying hospitality and hotel management at Hong Kong University; he was twenty-four and working on his PhD in statistics. His thesis was on the methodology behind the Hong Kong population census, and I needed data for a paper I was writing on disposable income among the city's upper class. He was quiet and well mannered, with piercing eyes that seemed to foreshadow a brilliant future, and he had a passion for numbers. But he didn't need to become a doctor in statistics or end up here in this country. He came from a Chinese family that over three generations had amassed wealth and influence helping the British authority administer the port of Hong Kong, and he had a high post guaranteed for him there. But he saw being associated with the "empire" as old-fashioned, even slightly dishonorable. Waiting for China's takeover of the administration of Hong Kong, which was on the horizon, was equally unappealing: he considered himself a free man and an anticommunist. He would say to me, 'I have my atheism in common with the communists, and that's all.' And I would say to him, 'No, you're not an atheist; you love statistics too much. You worship numbers.'

"We covered a lot of ground in that first meeting, which he suggested we hold at the racetrack cafeteria near the university. We did not, however, get to the census data I wanted, so we met again. And again. And again. We talked about everything: his British-style aristocratic upbringing and my modest rural roots; his rational, scientific mind and my more creative side; his infatuation with America and . . . mine, too! Yes, we had that in common: a naïve, idealized notion of America, as well as the undeniable beginnings of an attraction to one another.

"But while he was well on his way to experiencing America firsthand—he had job offers from universities in Las Vegas and Salt Lake, and an approved work visa—I had no real hope of ever making it there myself. Half jokingly, 'so that we can continue dating,' as he put it, he proposed that we should marry—I had no other way of obtaining a visa. And so we did, against strong objections from his family, who wanted him to marry within his class.

"He leaned heavily toward Salt Lake and felt it was the better offer by far, but he left it up to me to pick where we went. 'I'm dragging you there, so you decide,' he told me. Well, he wasn't 'dragging' me at all, because I was all too happy to leave. I wanted to experience America, and I wanted to be with him. So I had a decision to make, and as I had heard such miraculous things about Las Vegas in every hospitality course I ever took, I decided we would make it our new home."

🁫 🀱 🁫

"We were two newlywed Chinese kids in sin city, and we thought we were discovering America." As she said these words, Mrs. Kuong sighed and shook her head at what seemed like a long lost innocence. "We had only ten days before his job started, and fifty must-see casinos. In our simple minds, it was like visiting the fifty states, and we checked every casino we saw off our to-do list. In each of the fifty casinos, we forced ourselves to engage in what we thought were quintessential American traditions: we always ate in sports bars that broadcast baseball games, when neither of us knew the rules of baseball; I always ordered a hamburger with curly fries, when I really didn't like how curly fries seemed to absorb so much more oil than regular fries; and whenever a waitress dressed in a playboy bunny costume asked him what he wanted to drink, he always ordered bourbon, which he never drank—he never could tolerate alcohol, bourbon or any other type, because of that genetic mutation some Chinese people are born with, where you don't have the enzyme you need to metabolize liquor.

"So we were like casino parasites, doing our duty as honeymooners with a list of attractions to see in a city we thought was a microcosm of our host country, but we only rarely actually gambled. And when we did gamble, it was I playing the slot machines as he stood nearby rooting for me and lecturing me on the statistics of winning big—extremely improbable, he calculated, with the confidence of a newly tenured professor of statistics. Yet, even without feeling the need to gamble, he seemed to genuinely enjoy the hours we spent together in these casinos. He said the lights were pleasurable for him and he enjoyed watching them flicker. As for me, I enjoyed watching their reflection in his eyes."

With that, Mrs. Kuong turned toward her husband as though to check for any remaining glimmer in his eyes but only found a mask-like face transfixed on his lap, where his clenched fists were resting.

"And then he started gambling," Mrs. Kuong continued, turning to address me again. "I will never forget the first time I saw him sitting at a slot machine, about six months after our move to Las Vegas. I had taken a job as the banquets coordinator at a new casino, and I was walking out to have lunch with my manager. As I passed the main casino floor, my eye caught an Asian male—my husband!—sitting in the center of a cluster of slot machines on the casino's main floor. It was early in the afternoon, and I knew he taught a statistics course at that time. I asked him what brought him to the casino, and whether he was OK. He said his class was canceled, so he decided to surprise me by showing up for lunch but never made it to my office because he was distracted by the slot machines. He asked me what time it was and whether I was hungry. I told him it was two o'clock and invited him to join my manager and me for lunch. 'Two o'clock!' he gasped. 'I can't believe I've been sitting in this chair for three hours. Time just flew! Come to think of it, my arm is really hurting.'"

Pathological gambling is an impulse control disorder recognized in the DSM-IV. It affects between 1 and 2 percent of the general population but seems to be increasing at a faster rate among women, adolescents, and adults over sixty-five. Its core features include a strong urge to gamble and withdrawal-like symptoms when the person tries to abstain from gambling. To meet DSM-IV criteria for the diagnosis, one must have failed to cut back on gambling or suffered serious negative consequences as a result. These significant complications define *pathological* gambling as a clinical diagnosis and distinguish it from *social* gambling—the pleasurable pastime of an adult "who can take it or leave it." The DSM-IV criteria for pathological gambling disorder are listed on page 112.

"And so it went. From gambling when his class was canceled to canceling his class to go gamble, the problem gradually worsened and with it our financial situation. We were lucky initially, because

A. Recurrent gambling behavior characterized by five or more of the following:

    1. the person is preoccupied with gambling or gambling-related problems (e.g., reliving past gambling experiences, thinking of ways to obtain money with which to gamble, etc.);

    2. needs to gradually increase the wager amount to achieve the same level of excitement;

    3. has failed to control or stop gambling;

    4. is restless when attempting to cut back on gambling;

    5. gambles as a way to escape negative moods like depression;

    6. often returns after losing to "get even";

    7. lies to loved ones, therapists, and others about the extent of the gambling problem;

    8. has committed illegal acts like forgery, embezzlement, or fraud to finance his gambling;

    9. has seen personal relationships, work, or academic performance suffer as a result of gambling;

    10. relies on money from others to relieve gambling-related debt.

B. The gambling is not better accounted for by another psychiatric problem, such as the manic phase of manic-depressive illness.

Source: Adapted from the *Diagnostic and Statistical Manual of Mental Disorders*, 4th ed. Washington, DC: American Psychiatric Press, 1994.

his family was willing to help. They thought it was expensive to begin a new life in the United States, especially Las Vegas, of which they had a glitzy and hence expensive notion. So they set up an account for us and replenished it regularly, no questions asked. But after two years, the questions began, first as muttered grumblings, then gradually loudening into provocative questions and accusations. Did you leave your family and a lofty position with the port authority to take a low-paying job in America? When are you being promoted? It's good being a professor in America, but do you think you can raise a family on title alone? Or is it your wife who's spending the money, compensating at our expense for growing up a poor peasant? And why isn't she pregnant yet anyway?

"Yes, they blamed me for much of our financial problems and for our childless marriage. He was timid in defending me, and I think I can understand why: we really needed the money, and there was no easy explanation he could give them. I was already working overtime in the banquets department, but we could barely pay our bills, and loan sharks were constantly calling our house. I was petite and pretty, and Asian girls were scarce in Las Vegas back then . . . A Thai girlfriend who worked in the VIP club on the casino floor told me she was making a lot in tips and said I should consider an evening job with her. And so I did.

"He did not object to my move to the casino floor; he had graduated from losing quarters in slot machines to playing blackjack, so he needed even more money. Many Midwestern tourists had never seen an Asian girl before, and they tipped me generously. They would specifically request my table—'Fortune Cookie's table,' they would say—and if my table was full, they just left! They liked the 'Fortune Cookie' persona, and management liked it, too, and before too long, I was being asked to 'escort' our high-rollers. Well, you know what 'escort' means . . . I told my husband—I couldn't do such a thing behind his back, and I wanted him to know where his behavior was leading us. Maybe I wanted him to feel a little jealous, too. But again he did not really object—how could he? He had moved by then from blackjack— a game of some skill—to high-stakes roulette, a game of pure chance, and he depended on me and my Midwestern clients for his daily fix and to keep his debtors happy."

There are over 1,200 casinos, card rooms, and bingo parlors in the United States today, luring gamblers in part by manipulating a basic principle of human psychology, *operant conditioning*. This is a theory of learning best articulated by B. F. Skinner, which specifies that a behavior's consequences lead to a change in the frequency of its occurrence. According to this theory, the organism is seen to *operate* on the world, and as it does so, it encounters incentives and disincentives that make it more or less likely to perform the behavior. *Negative reinforcers* (e.g., the child has his crayons taken away for fighting with his brother) discourage the behavior, whereas *positive reinforcers* (e.g., the child gets a gift for doing well on a test) encourage it.

Very consistent positive reinforcement, however, can lead to *extinction*, or disappearance, of the behavior, as parents who consistently shower their children with love and attention find out when their child starts taking his parents' devotion for granted and loses the incentive to behave well, leading the good behavior to become extinct. On the other hand, a variable, unpredictable rate of positive reinforcement is much more resistant to extinction and keeps the child trying hard to impress his parents. This is the basic psychological mechanism behind addiction to slot machines—and gambling in general. You may not win often, but your next win could be right around the corner, so if you don't pull the lever on the slot machine (or roll the dice or play that hand), you will never know, and you may miss out on the jackpot of the century!

Behavioral scientists also work for casino owners trying to extract money out of gamblers in ways that go beyond operant conditioning. Free drinks offered in many casinos relax your inhibitions and increase your bets. Consistent lighting masks the passage of time and makes you more likely to linger longer at the blackjack table. Congregating slot machines in one area gives the illusion that more bettors are winning. And if you do notice arm fatigue working the slot machines, then modern technology has the answer in the form of armless machines where you only have to push a button for an almost instantaneous win!

⚏⚏⚏

"Dr. A., Dr. A., did you watch the ten o'clock news last night?" Dawn asked me as she popped her head into my office between two morning patients, with a mix of urgency and anxiety in her voice.

"No, I didn't," I answered. "What did I miss?"

"Well, I don't want to tell you how to do your job, but did you make sure Mr. Kuong wasn't taking the drug Mirasex?" she asked.

"Well, first of all, I think you meant to say Mirapex, not Mirasex," I said, chuckling. "And, second, can you tell me what is prompting you to play doctor with Mr. Kuong in the two minutes I have between patients?"

Dawn proceeded to enter my office and, after comfortably seating herself, started elaborating on the reasons for her concern. "Well it's just that this drug, which I understand you give to old patients with Parkinson's, can cause them to gamble their life savings away at slot machines, to the point where some can't afford to stay in their retirement communities anymore!" she said. "And these are poor upstanding old people who had never gambled before!"

"I'm glad that this is making it into the public consciousness," I said, realizing where Dawn's concerns were coming from—an article published in a specialized medical journal that had caught the attention of the mass media. It wasn't a simple concept to explain in two stolen minutes between patients, but I knew Dawn well, and I knew she would simply not be able to function at full capacity until I allayed her fears about Mr. Kuong's medication regimen. I also knew that she was liable to call him and inquire directly about his medication regimen out of concern. So I laid down my last patient's chart without finishing the visit note I had started writing and tried to explain. "Parkinson's disease is a condition where part of the brain stops producing dopamine, a neurotransmitter that is important in body movements," I said. "The stiffness and tremor you see in Parkinson's patients is a result of insufficient dopamine. Mirapex and similar medications work by increasing dopamine levels in the brain, which helps the movement problems in people with Parkinson's. However, all addictive substances—heavy ones like heroin, cocaine, and amphetamines, but also caffeine, alcohol, and tobacco—seem to work in part by releasing dopamine in the so-called pleasure circuit of the brain. Well, it's starting to look like addictive *behaviors* like gambling may do that, too. So giving someone a medication like Mirapex, which increases dopamine, could potentially cause a behavior like pathological gambling to show up as a side effect."

"So you're saying that pathological gambling, like smoking addiction, is biological and has to do with dopamine?"

"In a sense, yes," I said. "Just as people can become addicted to substances like tobacco, they can become addicted to behaviors like gambling. And just as we can see biological changes happen in people's brains as they develop a substance addiction, we are starting to learn of biological changes that seem to happen in the brains of patients with behavioral addictions as well."

"So Mr. Kuong is not on Mirapex, right?" Dawn asked again, looking satisfied with my explanation but realizing that I had not answered her question.

"No, he's not," I answered emphatically. "The good news is that this side effect from Mirapex is rare. Personally, I have never seen it in my practice."

My reassurance to Dawn that Mr. Kuong's illness was not a result of some tragic drug side effect seemed to make her facial features relax a bit—but only temporarily. "So what happens if Mr. Kuong were to develop Parkinson's in his old age and had to take Mirapex or something like it?" she asked, looking worried again. "How much worse can his gambling get?!"

There is growing acceptance that pathological gambling disorder may have a biological basis, but definitive scientific data are still scarce and have to be evaluated carefully, in part because of the frequent presence of substance abuse among pathological gamblers, which can cloud research conclusions. But even when problems like substance abuse are factored out, scientists still see evidence of impairment in the pathological gambler's frontal lobes, the seat of decision-making in the brain. This is borne out in elaborate psychological testing that shows them to be unable to balance immediate reward against known long-term negative consequences.

Genetic studies provide more support for the biological roots of pathological gambling. A study that compared 1,874 identical twin pairs to 1,498 fraternal twin pairs showed a significantly higher percentage of identical twins in which both members have pathological gambling disorder. Since the environment cannot explain this discrepancy (fraternal and identical twins usually grow up in identical settings), the higher percentage seen among identical twins is likely a result of their identical genetic makeup, which is not shared by fraternal twins.

⊞⋯⊞

"For his sake, for our sake, I had to get us out of Las Vegas. Eight years after we landed there, my husband was depressed, broke, and newly unemployed after his department put him on administrative leave for absenteeism. His parents had stopped sending money, saying they would resume only if he left his barren wife. As for me, I was depressed, too, but I could not dwell on my problems: I still had fantasies of saving him, and that required a lot of work and planning.

"Why try saving him, you might ask? Why put up with this? Why not take up with one of my rich, divorced Midwesterner clients? It's simple: I still loved him. Love is crazy, you know. I think you call it psychosis in your business. Well, I had that disease. Add to this illness the wifely duties deeply ingrained in me by Chinese culture, and you may begin to understand why I opted to stay.

"But on top of all this, I also felt some guilt and some responsibility for what had happened to him. Remember, he didn't have to come to Las Vegas. I was the one who picked it over Salt Lake City, which had no gambling opportunities, even though he had a much better offer from Salt Lake. I made my decision somewhat selfishly, because I thought it would be a great opportunity for me to be part of Las Vegas's hospitality business. If I had taken us to Salt Lake instead, I probably would not have been seeking to relocate us eight years after arriving in America. Who knows, he might have even become the chair of his department by then, and I might have allowed myself to get pregnant and open my dream restaurant . . . Instead, eight years into our American adventure, what we saw when we looked in the mirror was a suicidal addict and a high-priced prostitute!

"But thanks to me, we were not completely without options. If you grow up poor, you learn to work hard and save a portion of whatever money comes your way. So while keeping him on a tight financial leash, I renegotiated and gradually paid off his loans. I still managed to set aside some money every month, with the idea of achieving my primary goal of moving us out of Las Vegas. When I had saved enough money, I thought of San Francisco. It sounded like a perfect place for a fresh start: sunny, hospitable to immigrants, and most importantly, devoid of casinos! Plus, its people have sophisticated palates, and I was finally ready to fulfill my other goal of opening a high-end Cantonese restaurant in this country.

"We moved to San Francisco in late 1997. Within two months, I had leased a space for our restaurant and hired the kitchen staff. I decided that I would take care of the front of the restaurant, handling customers and money, and he would oversee the kitchen.

I was fortunate to find a French-trained cook of Chinese descent who was able to precisely capture the style I had in mind for the place: cosmopolitan interpretations of traditional Cantonese dishes unknown to the American public, offered in a contemporary, clean space. Only six months later, a rave review by our powerful local food critic changed everything. 'Rediscover Chinese' and 'Thank you, Vegas, for letting the Kuongs go,' it read. Before long, I had to hire a reservationist to handle the onslaught of phone calls and the waiting list that followed the four-star status the critic bestowed on us. Throughout it all, I was happy to be doing something I believed in: introducing aspects of our culture to an appreciative audience that we respected, in a part of the country we loved. But mostly, I was happy to see my husband happy. He was a proud man again, finding meaning and a sense of accomplishment in what he was doing, and no longer preoccupied by his addiction. And when the urge to gamble did cross his mind, knowing he could not easily satisfy it in San Francisco somehow made it easier for him to ignore. His energy and attention shifted back to productive work and, to my surprise, to cooking. Within months, not only was he overseeing logistics of the kitchen but he was also counseling our chef on recipes, altering the braising temperature here, adding a new spice there, and all for the better! And that's coming from a man who had never boiled an egg in his life, who depended on his family cooks for food while growing up in Hong Kong and on me for everything after we moved here."

Collectively, gamblers in the United States lose over $80 billion annually, a figure that has grown every year for the last two decades, now surpassing combined entertainment and leisure returns from venues such as movie box office, spectator sports, recorded music, and cruise ships. Still, large as this number is, it does not include the billions lost in illegal gambling every year or in the largely unregulated Internet gambling business, now conducted out of an estimated 2,300 offshore-based Internet casinos.

But what do these staggering figures mean at the level of the individual pathological gambler? For many, their financial burden leads to spiraling depression, along with other negative consequences, including bankruptcy, divorce, substance abuse, and forensic repercussions from illegal activities that desperate gamblers sometimes resort to, such as theft, bad checks, and embezzlement.

One particularly ominous consequence is suicide. The rates of suicide are up to four times higher in cities with legalized gambling compared to similar cities that outlaw gambling. Las Vegas, the premier gambling destination in the United States, has the highest suicide rate in the nation, among both residents and visitors.

∎∎∎∎

"So, Dr. A., have you tried their restaurant yet?" Dawn asked after one of my appointments with the Kuongs. "I know they gave you a gift certificate last week."

"No, I sure haven't," I answered. "I find it a bit problematic, ethically, to accept their gift. Plus, I rarely feel like eating Chinese anymore. I don't know what it is."

"Yes, we rarely go out for Chinese ourselves, either," Dawn answered. "I guess Thai is our new Chinese."

"Then Vietnamese must be my new Thai," I said.

"You're always a step ahead," Dawn answered, pausing a bit before adding, "culinarily." Then, after another brief pause, she added, "Well, we made an exception and went out for Chinese yesterday. The Kuongs were generous enough to give me a gift certificate, too, and we decided to go—I hope it's OK!"

"It's rarely OK to accept gifts from patients, and we should only do it if we can be sure it won't influence treatment in unfair ways," I said. I wanted to discuss this important issue with Dawn in more detail, but my intense curiosity about her experience in the Kuongs' restaurant made me drop the subject. "How was it?" I asked.

"Well, it's no ordinary Chinese restaurant, that's for sure," Dawn said. "They call it Canton cuisine. No tanks of live fish swimming in green water greet you at the door there . . . Instead, you get an immaculate-looking Mrs. Kuong, smiling broadly as she welcomes you, wearing a flowing red dragon kimono, red satin slippers, and the brightest red lipstick you ever saw. I had to compliment her on her appearance, so I told her she reminded me of the delicate porcelain dolls I used to collect. She graciously thanked me, saying that she wore red for good luck, in keeping with Chinese tradition. And—silly me!—I had assumed that her red had something to do with growing up in communist China. In any event, Mrs. Kuong looked like a doll, but Hector, of course, had to disagree, which almost ruined our evening. He dared tell me after she seated us that he thought she looked like a hooker! Imagine! Our gracious hostess, Mrs. Kuong, a prostitute! Well, fortunately, he was quick to apologize, and we were able to get to our first course."

I was intrigued by Dawn's description and even more by Hector's intuitions. I knew from my meetings with the Kuongs up to that point that they were doing poorly and were contemplating moving again, but had no detailed information yet on how bad Mr. Kuong's symptoms now were or how they might be affecting his wife.

"It's hard for me to picture the whole scene," I said to Dawn. "It's so different from the context in which we usually see them . . . But tell me more. Did you actually see Mr. Kuong?"

"I did," Dawn answered. "He was helping in the kitchen, looking the way he normally does—passive and subdued. He barely lifted his head out of the stock pot to acknowledge me when I snuck into the kitchen to thank him for the invitation."

"I'm sure he didn't mean to be disrespectful," I said. "As you can imagine, there's a lot on his mind. But did you at least enjoy the food?"

"Oh, the food was delicious," Dawn answered. "No Mongolian beef or Kung Pao chicken or sweet and sour pork there! Instead, you get 'a four-star symphony of flavors and textures,' as our paper's food critic said, and you know that man is always right! I just wish we could afford more of the places he recommends, but not on my clerk salary and with Hector slaving away for free at his Internet startup!"

"Well, Chinese cuisine deserves a stylish, creative outlet in our area," I said, "and I'm glad the Kuongs are filling the niche. But tell me, what was your favorite part of the meal?"

"Well, I liked it all," Dawn answered, "but I must say my favorite part came at the end, when Mrs. Kuong brought out an oversized fortune cookie on a silver plate for us to share. Again, not your mother's fortune cookie! This was more like a giant lacey shell with tiny sugar crystals that looked like pearls decorating the outside, and it just melted in your mouth!"

"All this talk about delicious food is making me very hungry; perhaps I should reconsider Chinese," I said. "One more question before I go get lunch: do high-end fortune cookies still come with a hidden message inside?" I asked, expecting the answer to be no—too pedestrian perhaps for the kind of restaurant this was espousing to be.

"They do, indeed," Dawn answered as she smiled at the memory of the flavor of the fortune cookie or the message inside the shell. " 'You will win big' is what ours said, which got Hector excited about his Internet start-up actually making it. Too bad they're not going public anytime soon!"

There are four major avenues for legal gambling in the United States: lotteries, charitable gaming, pari-mutuel wagering, and casino gambling. Lotteries have a colorful history that dates back to the early days of the North American colonies, when they were used to raise money for the operation of the new settlements. However, scandalous stories of fundraising abuses and profiteering eventually led to their banning from 1894 until 1964, when they were brought back in the form of the New Hampshire Sweepstakes. From New Hampshire, state-sponsored lotteries quickly spread to other northeastern states before crossing westward in the early eighties. Currently, multistate lotteries are the norm, with the large number of tickets sold allowing for larger jackpots.

Charitable gaming is operated for the benefit of nonprofit organizations; bingo and church raffles are its most common examples. Charitable gaming is the least regulated area of legal gambling; for that reason, it has come under criticism in several states for problems relating to fraud and accounting irregularities.

Pari-mutuel wagering, from the French words for mutual betting, is a system where bets are made on competitors finishing in a ranked order. All money is placed in a pool and then divided among the winners, after deducting a house take and taxes. Common examples of pari-mutuel wagering include horse racing and greyhound racing.

Casino gambling accounts for the largest segment of the gambling market. Casinos are characterized by the offering of banked games such as slot machines. In banked games, the house acts as a participant and, as such, has a stake in who wins; this stands in contrast to nonbanked games, such as lotteries, where the operator has no such stake. In 1931, Nevada became the first U.S. state to legalize unlimited-stakes casinos. However, since the late 1980s, there has been a rapid increase in commercial casinos that offer banked games. Initially, these casinos were regulated, either by capping the stakes or by restricting them to settings such as riverboats, which gave the illusion of containment and control. However, there seems to be an inexorable nationwide movement toward relaxing these limitations, both by removing the cap on wagers and by moving the physical address of the casino, in stepwise fashion, from the waterway, to dockside, and finally to land.

⬚⋯⬚

"I still remember my excitement filling out my first ballot in November 1998," said Mrs. Kuong. "We had just been sworn in as U.S. citizens, and I was thrilled to be voting for the first time. Our restaurant had just made it into the top-five category based on a large survey of restaurant goers, and everything seemed stable and promising. I hadn't done my homework before voting, and in my elated state in the voting booth, I almost missed Proposition 5, hidden as it was under the innocent-sounding 'Economic Self-Sufficiency' title. But when I read the small print, I understood that it aimed to bring gambling to California. No, this could not be happening to us, I thought to myself! Not now, not again! In a flash, I saw our new life taken away from us, my husband returning to gambling, our restaurant losing customers and stars, and me going back to bailing him out any way I could. I quickly checked no on Proposition 5, leaving the rest of the ballot blank, then walked out of the voting booth, deeply disappointed with my first taste of democracy."

The spread of gambling in the United States over the last decade has been largely driven by the exponential rise in Indian gaming, revenues from which reached $20 billion in 2004. At play in the passionate debate around Indian casinos are many legitimate but often divergent issues, including the right of a marginalized community to self-governance and economic revival, the need of cash-strapped states for tax revenues and job opportunities, the public interest in a safe and regulated gambling environment, and the realization that, for a sizeable proportion of individuals, increased access to gaming inevitably leads to increased uncontrolled gambling, with all the personal, social, and criminal consequences this entails.

Initially, several Indian tribes used their unique position as sovereign entities within the United States to start pushing, on Indian land, controversial games such as high-stakes bingo, then illegal under most states' laws. By 1988, it was clear that Congress had to weigh in on a debate being fought across the country, often polarizing communities. The resulting Indian Gaming Regulatory Act (IGRA) of 1988 set the terms for how Indian tribes could run casinos and bingo parlors by requiring a tribe-state dialog and a

binding contract between the two sides on how gaming opera-
tions should be conducted.

The California example is representative of this complicated
state-by-state battle. Failure to reach the IGRA-required agreement with one tribe led it to qualify Proposition 5, the Tribal
Government Gaming and Economic Self-Sufficiency Act, for the
November 1998 ballot. Voters overwhelmingly approved it, but
the state's Supreme Court struck it down in 1999. Another initia-
tive to allow Indian gaming, Proposition 1A, followed on the
March 2000 ballot, passing by a two-thirds majority. Despite
court challenges, Proposition 1A was upheld, leading to a mush-
rooming of Las Vegas–style casinos across the entire state. Currently, over forty-three tribes in California host some form of
gambling, and hundreds more are petitioning for Indian tribe status for purposes of building casinos.

Collectively, these casinos generate over $5 billion annually,
bringing great prosperity to a relatively small proportion of Na-
tive Americans. This prosperity translates into real political muscle; Indian tribes have become the largest contributor to California political campaigns.

⊡⋯⊡

"Proposition 5 got tied up in legal red tape, giving us a little
breathing room," Mrs. Kuong explained, "but then, in 2000,
came Proposition 1A, which passed by 65 percent. *Sixty-five percent!* Almost enough to make me miss communist China! I knew
that more legal wrangling would delay the appearance of casinos,
but I couldn't chase a growing worry out my mind: our lives had
become tenuous again, and all we had built together since leaving
Las Vegas was once again at risk.

"By early 2002, the democratic process had fully unfolded, and our first local casino opened, a mere ninety-minute drive away. I confronted my husband about my deep fears and asked him whether it was time to move to a safer place, but he reassured me that gambling was a thing of the past and that California was meant to be our home.

"Well, I should have known better than to share my husband's confidence in his self-control. By mid-2002, he was again so pre-occupied with gambling that he was overcooking the abalone in the kitchen. By late 2002, he was leaving the stove on in his rush to drive off to the nearest casino after work."

Several types of psychotherapy have been proposed for the treatment of pathological gamblers. The *psychodynamic* school sees gambling as a desire for self-punishment in someone who believes he has committed shameful mistakes. According to this model, therapy must uncover and resolve the roots of this guilt so as to obviate the need for self-flagellation. Few present-day therapists adhere to this model.

The *cognitive* model of psychotherapy attempts to challenge the faulty thinking that allows gambling behavior to persist. Faulty thoughts that I look for and try to confront in the gamblers I treat include selective recall of winnings, selective amnesia regarding losses, a belief that they possess special skills that make them more likely to win, and superstitions around fate and destiny.

A *behavioral* therapist helps the pathological gambler recognize sights, sounds, physical sensations, and a depressed mood that have become directly linked in his mind to gambling. In therapy, I try to uncouple these experiences from the gambling behavior, so one does not necessarily lead to the other. Thus the next time my patient feels depressed, it should not automatically lead to the nearest casino. Other behavioral changes I encourage my patients to adopt include having their paycheck go directly to their spouses, hence making money less accessible, and joining the self-exclusion lists that some casinos maintain to help gamblers "ban" themselves from a casino for a specified length of time.

Gamblers Anonymous is a popular twelve-step program modeled on Alcoholics Anonymous (AA) that I also frequently recommend to problem gamblers. It is free and widely available, with over a thousand chapters in the United States alone, and can be an important component of the treatment strategy. As in AA, participants in Gamblers Anonymous are encouraged to admit their powerlessness over their gambling problem and to invoke a higher power to help them conquer this problem. They are encouraged to seek support from their peers and from an assigned sponsor in overcoming their habit and to make amends to loved ones whom their gambling behavior has harmed.

❖❖❖

"Can you quantify for me, Dr. A., the response rate and the risk of side effects for this medication you are recommending, naltrexone?" This was probably the first meaningful complete sentence Mr. Kuong had uttered in my presence since our meetings began, and it came almost as a jolt. Until then, his wife had done all the telling and much of the emoting, with Mr. Kuong listening passively, very rarely indicating a reaction by shaking his head, tensing his facial muscles, or half-smiling.

But before I could answer his question, Mr. Kuong added, "It is hard for me to see how a simple pill can treat a behavior as complex as gambling. Not that I want you to recommend the talking cure, mind you—you've seen how talkative I am!"

Mr. Kuong was right in that I was not thinking of therapy for him yet, precisely for the reason he had sarcastically alluded to: his pronounced passivity and the difficulty he would have engaging in a productive and interactive therapy exchange. Mrs. Kuong, on the other hand, would have made an ideal therapy candidate; she was an articulate storyteller who was willing to look inward to explore the narrative behind things and then look outward for opportunities to do her therapist-assigned homework and apply her therapy-learned tools. I imagined her benefiting from therapy on several fronts, such as getting support in dealing with the frustrations around her husband's relapse, assuaging her guilt for exposing him to the environment that had brought about the gambling, protecting herself from his family's blame, and developing a better understanding of her taking up prostitution—an understanding that would go beyond the obvious financial motivations to explore any deeper, implicit desires for revenge or even self-expression. All these seemed like the kinds of problems for which therapy was invented, and she stood a good chance of benefiting from intervention, except that Mrs. Kuong was not my patient, and while I could strongly recommend therapy for her—and I did—it wasn't my role to be her therapist.

But it *was* my role as her husband's doctor to fully address his question, although I came up short when I tried to martial specifics and statistics to bolster my medication recommendation. "I wish I could tell you exactly what the response rate and the risk of side effects are," I said, "and I can understand why the statistician in you would demand precise numbers. Unfortunately, the studies done so far are too small for us to be able to generalize the data in a confident manner. One reason I'm recommending naltrexone, though, is because there is more data that suggest it can be helpful for some people. Unfortunately, however, the data also indicate that it carries a small risk of liver irritation. With good monitoring of your liver through blood tests, though, we should be able to catch any liver damage relatively early, should it occur, and be able to stop it."

Mr. Kuong shook his head in disagreement and appeared to be preparing to persuade me to change my recommendation, although I don't know to what. Before he could verbalize anything, however, an exasperated Mrs. Kuong stood up, turned toward her husband, and wagging her finger at him, loudly interjected, "Whatever the response rate is, it is higher than the likelihood of you coming out of this on your own. And whatever the risk of damage to your liver is, it is less than the risk of our restaurant losing a star, or us going bankrupt, or me finding another husband!" Then, regaining her seat and sounding more resigned than angry, she added, looking at me this time, "But I also have to be realistic and consider the possibility that nothing will work. So, while I want him to take the naltrexone, I have to continue to pursue what worked last time—moving. Although we are running out of cities to move to as casinos spread, we will always have Salt Lake! In fact, I just got back from a trip there, and I think I've identified a restaurant space that would work: spacious, bright, and with a liquor license, which is no small feat in Salt Lake! Most importantly, though, it is nowhere near a casino. He will be flying there soon to look at it, too."

<hr />

Medications can play a role in the treatment of pathological gambling. The SSRIs have been the most studied drug class. Among them, paroxetine seemed promising based on early results, but a sixteen-week double-blind placebo-controlled study in seventy-six subjects showed no advantage over placebo.

Given its efficacy in treating alcohol addiction, naltrexone, a medication that blocks opiate receptors in the brain to which morphine binds, has been studied in behavioral addictions as well, including pathological gambling. Some researchers have speculated that blocking opiate receptors might work by interrupting the brain's pleasure circuitry. It is hypothesized that this might reduce the thrill associated with the addiction, making it easier to resist. In one eleven-week double-blind placebo-controlled study involving eighty-three volunteers with pathological gambling disorder, 75 percent of subjects on naltrexone improved significantly, compared to only 24 percent on a placebo. Unfortunately, a small fraction of patients on naltrexone may develop liver problems as a side effect, necessitating regular blood draws to monitor liver function.

"We got these from the lab this morning." Dawn sounded anxious as she handed me the results of Mr. Kuong's liver function tests, done five weeks after initiating naltrexone. "They don't look too good."

Dawn was right. Several liver enzymes had increased significantly from baseline levels drawn before starting the medication. There seemed to be only one explanation: Mr. Kuong had indeed developed the rare side effect.

"Let's get them on the phone," I said to Dawn. "He needs to stop the medication immediately, and we need to follow his liver enzymes daily to make sure they normalize."

"I hope it's OK, but I already talked to them!" Dawn answered. "You were back-to-back this morning, and I thought this couldn't wait, so I called Mrs. Kuong at the restaurant. She asked me if I wanted to hear the good news, and I said that I unfortunately had some bad news, and that I should go first, and she said to go ahead, so I told her about the blood tests and that her husband should probably stop the medication immediately. I then asked her for her good news, thinking that maybe the restaurant had won another star—"

"And what was the good news?" I asked Dawn. "Please don't tell me he had responded to the medication!"

"He had, he had, the poor thing!" Dawn said, tearing up and shaking her head in disbelief. "He hadn't been to a casino in three whole weeks! What are the chances?!"

We made sure that Mr. Kuong's liver irritation reversed itself, but the Kuongs decided not to start another medication for fear of side effects, and Mr. Kuong still adamantly refused therapy. Instead, the couple used this incident as an incentive to speed up their plans for moving to Salt Lake. At our last meeting, the Kuongs thanked me and said they would send me a postcard once they had reestablished themselves in their new home. However, about four weeks after I last saw them, instead of a sunny picture of Salt Lake's Temple Square, a letter arrived from Mrs. Kuong, sent from San Francisco.

Dear Dr. A.:

I feel broken writing this to you. What started out as two bright-eyed students falling in love at the racetrack cafeteria near Hong Kong University ended with one lonely man empty-ing a gun down his throat in a desolate hotel room in downtown Salt Lake.

In case details still matter at this point, my husband relapsed within two weeks of stopping the medication. At my insistence, he traveled to Salt Lake to view the restaurant space I had identified on my trip there. Well, what I did not realize is that casinos now come to you, so there is no longer any sense in trying to run away from them. According to the forensic report I obtained, the Internet browser on my husband's laptop was frozen on a gambling Web site, www.fortunecookie.net, and he appeared to be in the middle of a credit card transaction when he pulled the trigger.

I know that ultimately you were not able to help him, but I do not fault you for that. I know you did help *me*. Even as I say that I feel broken, I am not entirely without hope, and I think this is in part because I got to tell my story, first to you and then to another therapist I have started seeing at your recommendation. So thank you! But please allow me to say so in person, too. Please join me, with Dawn, for a dim sum memorial lunch at our restaurant on Saturday. In lieu of flowers, I'm asking that attendees donate to the ongoing campaign against Internet gambling.

Very sincerely,
Mrs. Kuong

The tribute over dim sum for Mr. Kuong was a moving, delicious, and beautifully orchestrated affair. Mrs. Kuong looked sad but also peaceful and almost angelic in her silk wrap dress, all in white, the Chinese color of mourning. As she walked among tables, depositing a white rose on an empty plate here, and offering seconds of *shiu mai* and *har gaw* dumplings there, she radiated serenity and graceful hospitality. In the way she paused, a bit longer than at the other tables, to refill a bowl of deeply aromatic congee soup for a man I recognized as our paper's powerful food critic, Mrs. Kuong also showed her intention to continue, alone, in the local restaurant business.

But as I took in the scene around me, I could not help but wonder whether other treatment decisions I could have made might have prevented this terrible outcome. Every psychiatrist knows there will be some patients he cannot help, whether because of some lack of skill or empathy, because the patient is not ready for treatment, or perhaps because some essential chemistry is missing in the doctor-patient relationship. My failure with Mr. Kuong nagged at me every day and disrupted my sleep at night. So much of life depends on chance. I could not help wondering, what if Mrs. Kuong had taken her husband to a psychiatrist in a different city, perhaps Las Vegas? What if she had picked a psychiatrist who shared their culture and spoke their language? Would Mr. Kuong be alive today? Could someone else have helped him in a way I did not?

In the midst of this guilty soul-searching, I suddenly remembered a statistic I read once (but was a bit too superstitious to verify!): 50 percent of psychiatrists lose a patient to suicide in the course of their professional lives. This recollection sent me deeper into negative thinking and left me feeling distinctly unlucky. Why did I have to join this somber half so early in my career? I remember comparing how crushed I felt then with how detached and secure in my own abilities I was when I first read the statistic. I also remember thinking that, with any luck, perhaps I had met my sinister "quota" as a psychiatrist, and this would never happen to another patient of mine.

One Eternity Drive

In retrospect, it should not have taken a comprehensive psychiatric interview or the battery of tests I put my patients through to understand Alex's problem. Dawn could have accurately diagnosed him from three e-mails she received from him—and forwarded to me—in quick succession one morning. The first one read:

Dawn,

You must have reviewed with the doctor by now the phone screen you did with me yesterday. Please e-mail me at your earliest convenience to set up an appointment with him. It's 8 A.M. now.

Alex

At 8:15, he wrote:

Dawn,

Still no sign of life from your clinic . . . I'm really eager to see the doctor and get evaluated.

Anxiously waiting,
Alex

By 8:30, Alex was clearly desperate:

Dawn,

If it's difficult to set up an appointment with the doctor for a
face-to-face evaluation, can he perhaps e-mail me his questions?
I can e-mail my answers back, and he can give me his recommendations. Better yet, can you please check whether he would
meet me in a chat room? Don't worry! I can set it up so we have
total privacy.

Alex

Dawn attached her commentary to the last forwarded e-mail:

Dr. A.,

Would you ask this guy to log off already? "Can you please
check whether he would meet me in a chat room?" Yeah, right!
And maybe I can start telecommuting to clinic and checking
people into chat rooms from the comfort of the kids' playroom.
Unbelievable!

Dawn

Despite its relatively young age, the Internet has radically and ir-
reversibly changed many aspects of how we work, play, learn, and
express ourselves. According to estimates by the Nielsen/Net
Ratings Web site, U.S. Internet household penetration reached
75 percent in early 2006, with the number of active users still
growing and the speed of Internet connections continuing to rise.
Many advantages lure users to the Internet. These include the

convenience it adds to a wide spectrum of basic tasks, from paying
utility bills to buying movie tickets; the sheer breadth of the information it makes accessible, overshadowing all other resources;
the chance to build communities, including the ability to connect
with people who share our interests, no matter how rare or nar-
row these interests might be; and, finally, the anonymity it gives
and the attendant freedom to express views or play out (usually)
harmless fantasies in front of a large audience in a way that is normally repressed by societal norms and constraints.

However, a dark side to this vast new world of opportunities has
emerged. Accumulating data point to individuals for whom the Internet becomes a consuming habit that takes over their lives, ex-
acting a significant toll along the way. Some of these individuals
are approaching psychiatric clinics across the country for help in
controlling the compulsion to use the Internet or dealing with the
aftermath of a destructive Internet habit. For lack of an established
diagnosis or an agreed-upon phrase to describe this phenomenon,
I will refer to these individuals as *problematic Internet users* and will
call the clinical condition *problematic Internet use.*

A week later, Alex and I met for our intake appointment—held,
as all my sessions had been up to that point, face-to-face—in my
cramped office in our clinic building, an edifice made all too real
by overheating problems in the summer and occasional water
leaks in the winter.

"I don't consider myself to have an addictive personality," Alex
began. "I don't drink or do drugs. I don't get addicted to the kind
of habits that bring people to this clinic, either: I don't check or
clean excessively; I've never gambled; and I don't pick my skin or

pull my hair or bite my nails compulsively. But I'm an addict nonetheless. A modern-day addict.

"For as far back as I can remember," Alex continued, "I've been extremely shy. Whenever I could, I minimized my interactions with people. I built my few friendships by carefully socializing in small groups and even made career choices that limited random, spontaneous run-ins with people—that is how I became a research physicist working with radioactive isotopes under strict isolation. But one area where I could not accommodate my anxiety was dating. I still had to put myself in unfamiliar situations where I might meet a new girl, then muster the courage to ask for her phone number, then find it in me to actually call her, and then make it to our first date without canceling at the last minute for some made-up excuse. After countless false starts that kept me celibate until twenty-nine, a therapist finally recommended online dating. It was a good way to 'break the ice,' she said, because online personals ensured that basic compatibilities were met and thus reduced the likelihood of a complete mismatch, with all the stress that would entail. Once a posted profile catches your eye, the low-pressure e-mail exchange that follows allows you to learn more about the person, and to do it from a comfortable distance. If after this e-mail back-and-forth you still like the woman on the other side of the screen, you can arrange a first meeting, feeling like you 'know' her, which reduces the anxiety considerably. And so, at age thirty, after a two-month e-mail courtship, I finally met my first girlfriend, Nadia—I mean, Natalie.

"So the Internet allowed you to start dating, in part by helping you overcome paralyzing social anxiety," I recapped for Alex. "What went wrong?"

"It all started rather insidiously," Alex began. "Until I used the online dating service, I had used the Internet mostly for work-related e-mail and for searching the scientific literature. But with my dating profile posted for the world to see, I started feeling like I had to check it several times a day, sometimes several times an hour, to see how many hits it was getting. Were any responses waiting for me in my inbox, or even 'winks' from potentially interested women who could not take the time or, like me, were too anxious to write a full e-mail response? And how about Web sites that these women list in their profiles as being their favorite places to lurk online? I had to check those, too, since they could tell me a lot about them. And of course every time I went online I had to check for any new profiles that had been posted since the last time I logged on, because I wanted to be the first guy to 'wink' at a girl I might be interested in. And so on. So you can see how by the time I met Natalie in person, I was spending three hours a day on unnecessary Internet browsing."

"But then you met Natalie," I said, "so I imagine you had less need to be online, assuming, of course, you liked her."

"Oh, I liked her," Alex said. "I liked her a lot. But, to my surprise, meeting her didn't reduce my time online. I simply shifted from personals to twenty or so blogs that I started following compulsively after they were recommended in some of the profiles I visited on the dating Web site. But I can't say that, even with this much time wasted daily, the Internet was interfering with my work or my relationship with Natalie back then. We still progressed happily through the normal stages of courtship: a few tester dates, a few intimate dates, some camping trips we took where I didn't have Internet access and where I certainly missed my blogs but was able to enjoy the trips anyway, meeting the in-laws, getting engaged, and finally planning to get married and starting the process of finding a house to buy together."

Then, as if to prepare me for information on the pathological state that had brought him to my clinic, Alex sat up in his chair, moving it closer to me. His voice took on a more serious tone as he added, "It was right around the time when we started talking seriously about marriage that I snuck online one Sunday afternoon, literally between open houses with Natalie, to check a favorite blog, only to be directed by the blogger to the Web site that would change my life: www.altlife.net."

" 'Alt' as in 'alternate?' " I asked.

"Yes," Alex replied. "It's an online community that advocates dropping out of normal life and living, virtually, whatever alternate existence you wish to have for yourself. There, your identity is yours to define and manipulate as you see fit, with no socioeconomic, IQ, or psychological barriers. So if you always wanted to be a doctor but your grades did not permit it, you can still, for a small subscription fee, become altlife.net's Dr. So-and-so. Similarly, if you wanted to be an Olympic athlete but were born with a clubfoot, deformity does not have to encroach on your dream. Just design your body, using the software they make available, to be disability-free. And—this is true of me—if you were plagued by social anxiety in your real-life interactions, you still have a chance to become the most outgoing, life-of-the-party character you can imagine. This is what inspired me to create Sasha, a gregarious, Maserati-driving jock type in his mid-thirties, who is CEO of an Internet start-up that he just took public, making millions in the process."

The description of Sasha seemed to bring out happier tones in Alex's voice and a luminous quality in his eyes. With evident excitement, he continued, "Using the site's graphics tools, I meticulously painted in Sasha's hair, golden streak by golden streak, and picked 'azure blue' to fill in the eyes and 'snow white' for his teeth. I paid extra for a fully loaded subscription to the Web site, and exchanged my credit in their Central Bank for zlottes, altlife.net's official currency. With my zlottes, I bought Sasha a prime piece of real estate on the edge of Lake Eternity with spectacular views over altlife.net's downtown. With my subscription level, I could pick whatever address I wanted for Sasha's residence, so I chose One Eternity Drive. I then spent months painstakingly building One Eternity Drive with my own hands using software."

I was surprised by the extreme turn Alex's story was taking and absolutely intrigued by this new, technology-enabled manifestation of the old pathology of reality-denial and evasion. "I can see, Alex, how such an active virtual life could conceivably take over one's real life," I said.

"It could take over one's real life," Alex interrupted, "or what we *call* real life. See, by then, I had started doubting the value of this life compared to the magnificent one I was creating for myself through this online persona. And gradually, the daily life I had always known, with its radioactive lab work, its real estate agents who won't leave you alone, and its chronic anxieties—*that* life became the alternate one. As I looked forward to checking, at least once an hour, Sasha's One Eternity Drive mailbox for messages from other residents, I let my mail at 4931 Post St., #135, pile up. And when faced with the choice of attending yet another open house with Natalie or going online to continue work on Sasha's house, there was no doubt that the latter was what I really wanted to do."

"I hesitate to pass judgment on the value of your online life," I forced myself to say to Alex in as neutral a tone as I could muster, "but it clearly does become a serious problem when it starts causing you and your loved ones pain and suffering." I added, "I imagine all this led to significant tension between you and Natalie, for instance."

"It certainly did," Alex answered, "but nothing like when I introduced her to Nadia."

"Nadia?" I asked, bracing for what other surprises Alex's story might yet bring.

"Yes, Nadia," Alex answered with a shy smile. "Nadia is an altlife.net resident I met online who then became Sasha's masterpiece girlfriend. With Nadia's permission, I perfected her features, freckle by freckle and eyelash by eyelash, all the while feeling the omnipotence of a Michelangelo. Nothing, Doctor, *nothing* had ever given me such power or such a euphoric high before. And the more time I spent online with Nadia, be it in movie theatres, having a quiet meal with her in Sasha's kitchen, or in bed, the more resentful Natalie became, understandably."

"Wait!" I interrupted, in disbelief over what I thought Alex was saying. " 'In bed?' You had sex with Nadia, an online character?"

"I did," Alex answered, "in the form of Sasha."

Given that a considerable amount of problematic Internet use likely happens in the wired workplace and on company time, the question of the economic impact of this behavior is a crucial one. As a slightly tangential example, Cyber Monday is gradually replacing Black Friday in the United States as the barometer of health for the holiday shopping season and hence for the overall economy. (Black Friday is the day after Thanksgiving, traditionally the busiest shopping day of the year, when consumers begin their holiday shopping; Cyber Monday is the Monday after Thanksgiving, when consumers start their online holiday shopping, largely on company computers.)

One gets a more meaningful hint of the toll on businesses of problematic Internet use by looking at the results of a published telephone survey. Of the 1,500 businesses contacted for the survey, 224 responded. Among respondents, 60 percent reported that they had disciplined, and over 30 percent had terminated, workers for excessive or inappropriate Internet use.

Some of these individuals ended up in our offices. For some time, we had been seeing in our Stanford clinic (located in Silicon Valley) people with problems relating to being disciplined at work for inappropriate Internet use or threatened with divorce at home because they could not "log off." We wondered initially whether this phenomenon was limited to our locale, with its exceptionally Internet-savvy population. Researchers in very different settings, however, notably Dr. Donald Black at the University of Iowa in Iowa City, had already identified a similar problem and published studies describing it. These early studies found the typical patient to be a thirty-something college-educated single white male who spent approximately thirty hours a week on Internet use that was not essential to his work or well-being, causing him significant distress and disability.

These studies, however, were too small to be representative, so our group designed a study to try to reach a wider sample of the population. To achieve our goal, we used a random-digit-dial telephone survey method and interviewed 2,513 adults. The survey was conducted in 2004 and covered all fifty states, in a manner proportional to the population in each state. The cooperation rate with the survey was 56 percent—a relatively good rate for telephone-based health-related surveys.

Given the lack of an established definition for this problem, we developed the survey questions by borrowing from diagnostic criteria for generally accepted psychiatric conditions that share features with problematic Internet use, such as OCD, impulse control disorders, and substance addiction.

Of respondents in our survey, 4 percent said they were preoccupied with the Internet when offline; 6 percent felt their personal relationships suffered as a direct result of the Internet; 8 percent went online on a regular basis to escape negative moods; 9 percent actively hid their nonessential Internet use from people around them; and 12 percent stayed online longer than intended on a regular basis. Of note, the average age of respondents was forty-eight; a similar study done in a younger cohort would very likely yield significantly higher rates across all survey questions, since younger people tend to be more Internet-savvy. Also, we did not use cellular phone numbers in this survey, which likely led to an underestimation of the problem, since problematic Internet users may be more likely to use cellular phones than landlines.

As in the earlier, much smaller studies, this survey was not designed to evaluate whether excessive Internet use was a symptom of other conditions, such as social anxiety disorder or major depressive disorder. For that reason, in patients whose relationship or work difficulties appear to stem from Internet use, it is crucial to rule out other clinical causes. For instance, is the patient spending excessive time online because he is paralyzed by social anxiety whenever he attempts to make contact with people or because he is too depressed to leave the house? In this scenario, focusing on "Internet addiction" risks ignoring serious and treatable conditions that are the root of the Internet problem. On the other hand, did the patient start out relatively free of depression and anxiety but still develop an Internet problem that then took over, leading to avoidance of social interactions and to depression? In this scenario, problematic Internet use might be a legitimate primary diagnosis. Because of all these confounders, which have yet to be elucidated, mental health professionals should generally try to avoid phrases like "Internet addict," which can be both dangerous to patients and harmful to our profession.

The media should also exercise some self-restraint when reporting on the issue in a manner that is wildly ahead of the science. Various media outlets have covered, with varying degrees of sensationalism, the subject of "Internet addiction," especially as it relates to online gambling and pornography. While it is praiseworthy to be opening the public's eye to a problem often lost in the positive glow surrounding the Internet, it is also dangerous to coin diagnostic terms and assign labels before rigorous scientific research fully justifies them. This research, unfortunately, is still in its infancy.

⊞∙∙⊟⊞

"I'm far from perfect, and I'll be the first to admit it," Natalie said at the outset of our meeting. "Like everyone else, I could stand to lose a few pounds, and I could be a bit smarter in life, although I don't think I would want to be too smart—it obviously didn't protect Alex from serious problems! And I could also come from a family that didn't carry early Alzheimer's in its genes . . . Maybe because of these shortcomings, I have unfortunately had a lot of practice with boyfriends breaking up with me. Most of them left me for other women, one for another man, and one even for the seminary! But never, Doctor, *never*, has a guy left me for an online picture before! Never has a guy left me for a bunch of pixels dancing on his screen, and never have I heard of such a thing happening to any other girl! Yes, Alex has decided to break up with me, Doctor. He says he wants to spend more time with Nadia, and that's playing quite a number on my self-esteem, as you can imagine. Being dumped for Nadia, when Nadia is nothing but an online character that he fashioned with software, is not something that even *my* thick skin can handle. God knows I am far from perfect, but one thing I am, Doctor, is *real*. I am *real*, Doctor!"

As she explained her impossible predicament, Natalie's voice grew loud with anger, and she yelled out "real" in a shriek capable of piercing cyberspace and reaching deep inside the pixelated walls of One Eternity Drive. I could not help but put my hand in hers in a comforting gesture, feeling the pulsating blood of this very real woman.

"I think you have tremendous qualities, Natalie, I really do," I said. "I want to do my best to try to be helpful, but I must admit that this is a new kind of problem that we mental health professionals are still learning how to address. However, I do have a plan of action that I will share with Alex at his next visit. For his sake and yours. Please take good care of yourself in the meantime."

▦ ⋯ ▦

"Pray for me, Dr. A.!" Dawn said, almost jumping with anxious excitement late in the afternoon, when normally a mix of fatigue and desperate tying up of loose ends defines that part of the workday for her.

"I don't think you've ever asked me to pray for you before," I said. "I hope it's for a worthy cause!"

"It is, for sure!" Dawn said. "We're finally going public tomorrow!"

"We are—I mean, you are?" I asked. "In 2006?"

"Yes," Dawn answered, "and all these years of working overtime will, God willing, soon be over. Yes, Hector's Internet start-up is finally having its initial public offering tomorrow! You didn't think it would happen, did you?"

"Honestly, no," I said, feeling guilty over my inability to muster up much excitement about Dawn's big day. "I thought the whole Internet IPO boom was behind us. It all sounds so, umm, late-nineties."

"Well, it *is* happening tomorrow," Dawn said, "and from what I hear based on early buzz, it's looking good! Well, maybe not enough-for-us-to-stop-working-tomorrow kind of good, but at least enough for us to afford separate bedrooms for the kids and for Hector to finally start drawing a real salary!"

"That's great, Dawn," I said, feeling more sad at the possibility of Dawn retiring from my clinic than excited at the ultimate realization of this family's American dream. "I probably know better than anyone else how hard you and Hector have worked and how long you have waited. I hope all this gets generously rewarded tomorrow. I won't promise to pray for you, but I will do a tribal dance in your honor or light a candle or something . . ."

"Thank you," Dawn answered. "You'll be the first to know if we hit the jackpot! I'll be here tomorrow morning, of course, but you'll forgive me if I'm a bit distracted or I have to leave a little early."

Then, looking more serious, Dawn added, "You know who needs a prayer more than I do, though? It's your patient Alex . . . Now, I'm no doctor, of course, but I've seen my share of suffering around here, and this is one sick kid! And his poor fiancée—she's so devastated she breaks my heart! Can we start *her* on something, too? Can you believe that, sick as he is, he's now refusing to schedule a return appointment? But if he thought for one second that Dawn would let him off easy—someone in such desperate need of help—he was wrong! So I tried to bring him back into treatment by resurrecting his old idea of meeting you in a chat room and guess what—he agreed to one more session. I thought this way we would at least get another chance with him. Just make sure you remember your password. It's *shrink*."

"Wait!" I said, incredulous and clearly behind, still stuck on processing the ramifications for me and my practice of Dawn "going public" the following day. "You decided . . . on my behalf . . . a chat room . . . a password . . . and *shrink?!*"

"Yes," Dawn replied. "You can't resist online medicine forever, Dr. A. It's the wave of the future. Just make sure you remember your password. *Shrink*."

Whether we medical care providers approve of the phenomenon or not, Internet-based communications are gradually eroding the office confines that have for so long defined the doctor-patient relationship. I already allow e-mail, for instance, for scheduling purposes, but increasing numbers of doctors are also starting to use e-mail to dispense advice on such subjects as symptom management and medication side effects. Our patients certainly routinely check our recommendations against the endless array of variable-quality advice available online, and sometimes use the Internet to search for whatever information they can find on us, too. As the reach of the Internet inevitably grows, it becomes more important to seriously explore the pros and cons of practicing online medicine (e-medicine), including, for mental health professionals, online therapy (e-therapy).

One can imagine e-therapy opening the door to much-needed treatment for desperate patients who otherwise would likely have to go without. Think, for instance, of psychiatric patients in remote areas underserved by mental health professionals, or patients whose symptoms prevent them from leaving the house (such as patients with OCD who have severe contamination fears), or patients who, in addition to their psychiatric problems, have physical disabilities that prevent them from making it to their therapists' offices. For such patients, an online counselor might constitute a true lifeline.

But e-therapy also comes with serious risks, some shared with other Internet-based interactions and some unique to the business of therapy. For example, so much of therapy happens through interpreting and reflecting back to the patient nonverbal cues given off during the therapy session. These include strategic pauses, surprised looks, meaningful head shakes, and grimaces. The absence of these useful cues online can lead to misdiagnosis and misunderstanding, and to difficulty analyzing transference and countertransference issues. The result might be a stunted therapy experience that lacks the usual cogs that help propel it forward.

And the impersonal nature of the online therapy exchange may prevent a true bond from forming between patient and e-therapist. Although the informal and anonymous nature of the experience may help patients feel more at ease divulging deeply embarrassing thoughts and feelings online, the therapy relationship is what really inspires patients to come back and to maximize the benefit from the experience.

Another complication is the unregulated nature of the e-therapy landscape, where psychiatrists, psychologists, social workers, marriage and family therapists, faith-based counselors, "life coaches," and uncertified "counselors" operate loosely in the absence of any real laws guiding the practice of e-medicine and with little clarity about who is licensed to treat whom and what insurance, if any, patients have against malpractice should things go wrong in this new experimental field.

Equally important are confidentiality concerns, a risk in any online interaction, but more so when mental health records are at stake. Some e-therapists have devised ways to ascertain the identity of the person behind the screen name, such as agreeing beforehand on a password the patient gives prior to initiating an online session or briefly conferring by telephone before each session. Other privacy pitfalls have yet to be resolved. Many Internet service providers (ISPs), for instance, automatically maintain complete records of all online exchanges that go through their servers. (In contrast, most traditional therapists keep only condensed summaries of their sessions with patients.) Whether such detailed online records enjoy the protection of traditional therapist-patient privilege, or whether they would have to be disclosed if requested during a malpractice suit, remains to be established.

I decided to conduct Alex's online session from home but approached my computer with unusual trepidation as I typed the Web address for altlife.net. Once on the homepage, I chose the name Doc for my guest registration and was given the option of either building my personal altlife.net body from a gallery of body parts or accepting a generic body. I chose to do the latter and followed the plentiful signs to guide my borrowed body to the Convention Center, where Alex was to be waiting.

I recognized Sasha immediately. The blond streaks and jock good looks that Alex had so carefully described gave him away.

"Hello, is this Alex?" I typed, as a bubble rose from my character's mouth with my words in a playful cursive script. "This is Dr. A."

"Hi! Thank you for coming all the way here," Alex answered. "Password, please?"

"Oh, of course," I typed. "It's *shrink.* Thank you for remembering to ask."

"Great," Alex answered. "Let's get started then. You've probably heard from Dawn that I've decided to drop out for a while and focus exclusively on my online life. I don't know where it will all eventually lead, but it feels liberating and strangely empowering for now to not have a fiancée or scheduled meetings or a regular job. I feel oddly at peace having made my decision."

"I don't want to judge, Alex," I said, "but don't you feel like you have crossed a dangerous line, that you are creating a complete rupture between who you are here and who you used to be?"

"I do feel like I have, Doc," Alex answered, "but much more than a clinical symptom, this has become a philosophical and spiritual quest for me. What is at stake in these chat rooms in my opinion is nothing short of the meaning of life itself, and what this community is engaged in is nothing if not a radical reconsideration of all the constraints and assumptions that our society continues to blindly accept."

"I appreciate the grander issues this brings up for you, Alex," I said, "I really do. But to think that you can fully answer them here is futile. Especially when you consider the cost! Look at everyone who tried to answer these questions before you and fell short. Look at the countless examples from philosophy and religion. To expect to resolve, on altlife.net, the fundamental problem of existence . . ."

"You're asking me to be defeatist about it," Alex interrupted, "to not even *ask* the question, because nobody has been able to answer it to your satisfaction before."

"No, Alex," I said, "but I *am* asking you to please keep a foot in both worlds. By all means, do reflect on the grander issues, and do it here if you want, but do it without completely withdrawing from a life where your existence, fraught as it was, still had meaning, lots of meaning. And do it in a way that doesn't hurt people I know you still care about. Natalie, for instance . . ."

A silence followed—I think—evidenced by an empty bubble that hung over Sasha's head for what felt like an eternity.

"Alex, are you there?" I asked.

"Yes," he responded. "I'm just thinking." After another long pause, Alex added, "Well, if I decided to accept your recommendation, how would I go about keeping 'a foot in both worlds,' as you put it?"

"Here's the approach I think we should take," I said with new optimism. "First off, I know that severe social anxiety has plagued you for your entire life, and this has made it difficult for you to feel completely at ease in real-life relationships and interactions. The good news about this disease, though, is that it *is* treatable with either medications or therapy, and I suggest we use both. Regarding your Internet life, I want us to better understand how you spend your time here before we start to gradually cut back on it. To that end, I will ask you to develop a detailed log of where you go online, and what you do and how much time you spend doing it. Then, I will ask you to rank your online activities in the order of how attached you are to them, from the most fulfilling to the least fulfilling. Once we have developed this list, I will ask you to slowly decrease your online time, starting with those experiences that bring you the least pleasure. And as we start cutting back on your online time, we will think of specific real-life activities you can enjoy instead to occupy this freed up time. Although these are uncharted waters, I really think that this is the right way to proceed and you will ultimately be happier for it."

How I wished I could read Alex's facial features for indications of how my suggestions were being received and whether I had any chance of saving him! But no such signals were available to me. After a lengthy silence, I added with some desperation, "And we can continue to meet online for now if you want, just like today! This is actually much less scary than I thought!"

The bubble over Sasha's head still did not fill up, creating what I can only describe as palpable tension in the chat room. Then, finally, Alex's words came hitting back: "I'm sorry, Doc, but I'm just not invested enough in this to try it out right now. I do appreciate your perseverance, though. Now, if I may, I have one last favor to ask of you. If she comes to see you, please help Natalie understand that I didn't mean to hurt her, and that I cannot totally control this. Thank you. I think I will log off now. Goodbye."

With that, Sasha disintegrated into infinitesimally small dots that were quickly incorporated into the chat room's dark background. Watching him slowly vanish, like a small cloud of milk in a cup of hot coffee, I felt a small piece of my professional self-confidence melt away, too, along with any doctorly savior fantasy I may have had about being able to help someone who is not yet ready to fully acknowledge having a problem, or who is not yet ready for change.

But I could not give up on Alex so quickly, so I lingered alone in the chat room, hoping he would log on again, maybe with a change of heart, perhaps a compromise, or even just a simple follow-up question. To kill time, I picked an appropriate face— "sad and forlorn"—for my generic body, using the pop-up menu available free of charge to altlife.net's visitors. I even started personalizing other details in my look, picking "walnut" for my hair color (close to my natural hair color) and "sea foam" for my eyes (far from my natural eye color). But Alex never rematerialized.

Another guest did make an appearance, though: a balding man with an older face on a younger body, preternaturally blue eyes, a long white beard, and dressed in a white bathrobe with white slippers.

"Hello," he said.

"Hello," I answered.

"You look sad and forlorn," he ventured. "Can I help you?"

"I'm OK, thank you," I responded. "I'm just recovering from a difficult conversation with someone . . . Not a big deal, really. I should get going."

"But you must not go yet," the man said before repeating, "you look sad and forlorn. Can I help you?"

"I'm Doc," I said, feeling a bit detained but also oddly touched by this stranger's insistence on helping another stranger. "Who are you?"

"I'm God," the man answered. "You look sad and forlorn. Can I help you?"

An electric jolt ran through my fingers, up my spine and into my cortex on reading the man's response, causing me to ricochet away from my desk, almost disconnecting my computer and logging myself off in the process. I had come to the chat room to try to save a patient only to find God . . .

But after the shock came the warm and oddly comforting thought that, even in this netherworld, there are people who purport to look after people. Strangely, I was tempted to ask God to make himself available to Alex, but realizing that basic confidentiality rules governing my doctor-patient relationship with Alex still applied, I decided to shelf that idea and hoped instead that fate would somehow bring the two men together.

"I'm already feeling better," I said. "Thank you." Still, I could not go without availing myself of God's precious offer to help, so I thought hard of what else I might ask of him.

"There *is* actually something you can do for me, if it is not asking too much," I finally added. "A very deserving coworker—a friend, really—has a big day today and stands to find out soon whether her and her husband's long years of hard work will be financially rewarded. She asked me to pray for her, but I am not very good at that. Would you consider saying a prayer for her on my behalf?"

"I am God," the man reminded me, feeling, I imagined, somewhat slighted. "God does not pray," he said. "God *intervenes!*"

"Oh, of course," I said, anxious at the possibility of having hurt God's feelings. "Would you kindly consider *intervening* for her, then?"

A long pause followed that seemed to confirm my worry that I must have inadvertently upset God, opening myself up to unthinkable retribution.

"What is your friend's name?" the man finally asked.

"Her name is . . . her name is Aurora," I answered, relieved at God's continued willingness to engage me.

"Nice name," the man said. "I will see what I can do."

With that, the man dissolved, from the head down, into infinitesimally small white specks that were quickly absorbed into altlife.net's dark background.

⁑⁑⁑

I had very little reserve left in me after my morning online session with Alex and my brush with God, and found it difficult to return to business as usual in my brick and mortar office that afternoon. But I knew I had patients already scheduled, and I also had to find out what had happened to Dawn.

The colorful balloons and flower arrangements in our waiting area already announced the news: Dawn appeared indeed to have struck gold. I looked hard but could not see her at first, surrounded as she was by fellow clerks who had descended on our offices from all the clinics in the building to congratulate their new heroine. With difficulty, I managed to make my way to the center of the crowd, past trays of Mexican wedding cookies and bottles of non-alcoholic "champagne." There was Dawn, half-smiling and half-crying, having her Miss USA moment, with a bouquet of flowers in one hand and in the other a cell phone through which she was getting from Hector the market-close estimate of their net worth.

"Dr. A.!" she gasped on seeing me. "You must have prayed long and hard for me! The IPO went much better than anyone could have predicted! I can't even begin to wrap my mind around the number Hector just gave me. I don't think a tribal dance or a candle would have done this!"

"I think your and Hector's hard work over so many years is what did it, Dawn," I said. "Congratulations!"

Dawn then led me through the crowd and into my office for a more private conversation. "It hurts me to say this, but you know what this means," she said as she sat down. "It will be the end of an era around here . . . Don't worry, though, I will make the transition as smooth as possible and will spend as much time here as I need to make sure the next person is properly trained."

"Don't tell me you're retiring now just because you can afford to do so!" I said to Dawn, feeling a heaviness in my heart about losing her that was not completely offset by my genuine joy at this well-deserved happy ending.

"I have to," Dawn replied. "Hector wants me to, and I want to as well. There's so much we have deprived ourselves of over the years. We feel like we have a lot of catching up to do. We haven't even taken the kids to Mexico yet. At least this year we can do more than wish we were there for Semana Santa—we really have to start teaching them the Holy Week traditions before it's too late. You don't understand—they're growing up without rituals, they're growing up without culture!"

Dawn appeared to miss the irony involved in bringing rituals— our clinic specialty—and their role in culture into our conversation. I wondered whether pointing this out to her might inject some levity into the conversation. I even wondered if Dawn was implying that by helping us stamp out pathological rituals she was somehow contributing to the acculturation of the world!

Before I could decide how to respond, however, Dawn added, "We also need to find a new house. I'm thinking something on Grand View Avenue . . . What do you think? Not too bad for your old clerk, huh? We could be neighbors!"

Dawn winked as she mentioned the street I lived on in San Francisco. But the prospect of having Dawn as neighbor still did not allay my anxiety about losing her in the clinic, where I selfishly wanted Dawn to continue, just as she had over many years and countless difficult situations, providing support and inspiration for patient and doctor alike.

"But you've always found this job very fulfilling," I objected. "Think of all the patients you have helped. Won't they suffer?"

Realizing, however, that my guilt-inducing maneuver was unlikely to work, I tried an ideological argument instead, despite having no grounds for believing that Dawn subscribed to that ideology. "Think of your feminist ideals!" I said. "How can you reconcile those with retiring on your husband's income?"

Then, flashing back to the housewives on my street, I added, "It really shouldn't matter that you would be the only female on Grand View Avenue who worked." Finally, seeing that none of the points I was making was likely to influence Dawn, I settled for "OK, would you at least consider working part time?"

As my speech rambled on to match my mounting anxiety, I could feel my own unhealthy lifelong compulsion grow stronger: I was finding it very difficult to resist biting my fingernails. So, between desperate pleas to Dawn, I raised my hand to my mouth and, with deliberate up-and-down and sideways jaw movements, bit off pieces of bothersome nails.

But a very stubborn hangnail would not come out, which increased my anxiety, pushing me further into my insane soliloquy. So, to crown my performance, I gave Dawn my unsolicited professional opinion. "Dawn," I said, "I think I know you well enough to feel comfortable saying this: you would be crazy to give up all semblance of a career just because you now happen to be a millionaire. *Crazy!*"

Dawn, with a gesture that I can only describe as maternal, then reached for my hand with the hangnail, gently pulling it away and pinning it against the arm of my chair. "I guess, in the end, we are all a little bit crazy," she said.

REFERENCES

PSYCHIATRY BY THE DUMPSTER

Abed, R. T., and K. W. de Pauw. 1998. "An Evolutionary Hypothesis for Obsessive Compulsive Disorder: A Psychological Immune System?" *Behavioural Neurology* 11(4):245–50.

Campbell, S., and G. Macqueen. 2004. "The Role of the Hippocampus in the Pathophysiology of Major Depression." *Journal of Psychiatry and Neuroscience* 29(6):417–26.

Diagnostic and Statistical Manual of Mental Disorders, 4th ed. 1994. Washington, DC: American Psychiatric Publishing.

Freud, S. 1995. *The Standard Edition of the Complete Psychological Works of Sigmund Freud.* London: Hogarth Press and the Institute of Psycho-Analysis.

Jenike, M. A. 2004. "Obsessive Compulsive Disorder." *New England Journal of Medicine* 350:259–65.

Koran, L. M. 1999. *Obsessive Compulsive and Related Disorders in Adults.* Cambridge: Cambridge University Press.

Rasmussen, S. A., and J. L. Eisen. 1992. "The Epidemiology and Clinical Features of Obsessive Compulsive Disorder." *Psychiatric Clinics of North America* 15:743–58.

Rosenberg, D. R., F. P. MacMaster, M. S. Keshavan, K. D. Fitzgerald, C. M. Stewart, and G. J. Moore. 2000. "Decrease in Caudate Glutamatergic Concentrations in Pediatric Obsessive-Compulsive Disorder Patients Taking Paroxetine." *Journal of the American Academy of Child and Adolescent Psychiatry* 39(9):1096–1103.

Saxena, S., A. L. Brody, K. M. Maidment, E. C. Smith, N. Zohrabi, E. Katz, S. K. Baker, and L. R. Baxter, Jr. 2004. "Cerebral Glucose Metabolism in Obsessive-Compulsive Hoarding." *American Journal of Psychiatry* 161:1038–48.

Saxena, S., and S. L. Rauch. 2000. "Functional Neuroimaging and the Neuroanatomy of Obsessive-Compulsive Disorder." *Psychiatric Clinics of North America* 23(3):563–86.

Schwartz, J. M. 1998. "Neuroanatomical Aspects of Cognitive-Behavioural Therapy Response in Obsessive-Compulsive Disorder: An Evolving Perspective on Brain and Behaviour." *British Journal of Psychiatry*, suppl. (35):38–44.

Wolff, M., J. P. Alsobrook, and D. L. Pauls. 2000. "Genetic Aspects of Obsessive Compulsive Disorder." *Psychiatric Clinics of North America* 23(3):535–44.

H₂O UNDER THE BRIDGE

Alexis, A. F., R. Dubba-Subramanya, and A. A. Sinha. 2004. "Alopecia Areata: Autoimmune Basis of Hair Loss." *European Journal of Dermatology* 14(6):364–70.

Bhatia, M. S., P. K. Singhal, V. Rastogi, N. K. Dhar, V. R. Nigam, and S. B. Taneja. 1991. "Clinical Profile of Trichotillomania." *Journal of the Indian Medical Association* 89(5):137–39.

Christensen, G. A., R. L. Pyle, and J. E. Mitchell. 1991. "Estimated Lifetime Prevalence of Trichotillomania in College Students." *Journal of Clinical Psychiatry* 52:415–17.

Christensen, G. A., and S. J. Crow. 1996. "The Characterization and Treatment of Trichotillomania." *Journal of Clinical Psychiatry* 57 (suppl. 8):42–49.

Christensen, G. A., T. B. Mackenzie, and J. E. Mitchell. 1991. "Characteristics of Sixty Adult Hair Pullers." *American Journal of Psychiatry* 148:365–70.

Diagnostic and Statistical Manual of Mental Disorders, 4th edition. 1994. Washington, DC: American Psychiatric Publishing.

Jenkins, J. R. 2001. "Feather Picking and Self-Mutilation in Psittacine Birds." *Veterinary Clinics of North America: Exotic Animal Practice* 4(3):651–67.

Koran, L. M. 1999. *Obsessive Compulsive and Related Disorders in Adults.* Cambridge: Cambridge University Press.

Rothbaum, B. O., L. Shaw, R. Morris, and P. T. Ninan. 1993. "Prevalence of Trichotillomania in a College Freshman Population." *Journal of Clinical Psychiatry* 54(2):72–73.

A GREEK TRAGEDY

Aboujaoude, E., N. Gamel, and L. M. Koran. 2004. "Overview of Kleptomania and Phenomenological Description of Forty Patients." *Primary Care Companion to the Journal of Clinical Psychiatry* 6(6):244–47.

Diagnostic and Statistical Manual of Mental Disorders, 4th edition. 1994. Washington, DC: American Psychiatric Publishing.

Goldman, M. J. 1991. "Kleptomania: Making Sense of the Nonsensical." *American Journal of Psychiatry* 148:986–96.

———. 1998. *Kleptomania: The Compulsion to Steal—What Can Be Done?* Far Hills, NJ: New Horizon Press.

Hollinger, R. C., and J. L. Davis. 2003. *2002 National Retail Security Survey Final Report.* Gainesville: University of Florida.

Koran, L. M. 1999. *Obsessive Compulsive and Related Disorders in Adults.* Cambridge: Cambridge University Press.

McElroy, S. L., H. G. Pope, J. I. Hudson, P. E. Keck, and K. L. White. 1991. "Kleptomania: A Report of Twenty Cases." *American Journal of Psychiatry* 148:652–57.

WITH ANY LUCK

Cavedini, P., G. Riboldi, R. Keller, A. D'Annuci, and L. Bellodi. 2002. "Frontal Lobe Dysfunction in Pathological Gambling Patients." *Biological Psychiatry* 51(4):334–41.

Christiansen, E. M. 1998. "Gambling and the American Economy." In *Gambling: Socioeconomic Impacts and Public Policy*, edited by J. H. Frey. Thousand Oaks, CA: Sage.

Clark, K. 2005. "Against the Odds." *U.S. News and World Report* 138(19): 46–50.

Diagnostic and Statistical Manual of Mental Disorders, 4th edition. 1994. Washington, DC: American Psychiatric Publishing.

Dunstan, R. 1997. "Gambling in the United States." Chap. 1 in *Gambling in California*. Sacramento: California Research Bureau. http://www .library.ca.gov/CRB/97/03/Chapt1.html. Accessed September 10, 2006.

Gerstein, D., S. Murphy, M. Toce et al. 1999. *Gambling Impact and Behavior Study: Report to the National Gambling Impact Study Commission*. Chicago: National Opinion Research Center.

Goodyear-Smith, F., B. Arroll, N. Kerse et al. 2006. "Primary Care Patients Reporting about Their Gambling Frequently Have Other Co-occurring Lifestyle and Mental Health Issues." *BMC Family Practice* 10(7):25.

Grant, J. E., S. W. Kim, M. N. Potenza, C. Blanco, A. Ibanez, L. Stevens, J. M. Hektner, and R. Zaninelli. 2003. "Paroxetine Treatment of Pathological Gambling: A Multi-centre Randomized Controlled Trial." *International Clinical Psychopharmacology* 18(4):243–49.

"Growth in Indian Gaming." *National Indian Gaming Commission*. Available at http://www.nigc.gov/TribalData/GrowthinIndianGaming Graph19952004/tabid/114/Default.aspx. Accessed September 10, 2006.

"Indian Gaming in California." 2004. Institute of Governmental Studies Web site. Available at http://www.igs.berkeley.edu/library/ htIndianGaming.htm. Accessed September 10, 2006.

Kim, S. W., J. E. Grant, D. E. Adson, and Y. C. Shin. 2001. "Double-Blind Naltrexone and Placebo Comparison Study in the Treatment of Pathological Gambling." *Biological Psychiatry* 49(11):914–21.

Koran, L. M. 1999. *Obsessive Compulsive and Related Disorders in Adults.* Cambridge: Cambridge University Press.

Ladouceur, R., C. Sylvain, C. Boutin, and C. Doucet 2002. *Understanding and Treating the Pathological Gambler.* Hoboken, NJ: John Wiley and Sons.

Phillips, D. P., W. R. Welty, and M. M. Smith. 1997. "Elevated Suicide Levels Associated with Legalized Gambling." *Suicide and Life-Threatening Behavior* 27:373–78.

Potenza, M. N., H. Xian, J. F. Scherrer, and S. A. Eisen. 2005. "Shared Genetic Contributions to Pathological Gambling and Major Depression in Men." *Archives of General Psychiatry* 62(9):1015–21.

Reynolds, G. S. 1975. *A Primer of Operant Conditioning.* Glenview, IL: Scott Foresman.

Shaffer, H. J., M. N. Hall, and J. Vander Bilt. 1999. "Estimating the Prevalence of Disordered Gambling Behavior in the United States and Canada: A Research Synthesis." *American Journal of Public Health* 89(9):1369–76.

Stocchi, F. 2005. "Pathological Gambling in Parkinson's Disease." *Lancet Neurology* 4(10):590–92.

Winters, K., R. Stinchfield, and J. Fullerson. 1993. "Patterns and Characteristics of Adolescent Gambling." *Journal of Gambling Behavior* 9:371–86.

ONE ETERNITY DRIVE

Aboujaoude, E., L. M. Koran, N. Gamel, M. D. Large, and R. T. Serpe. 2006. "Potential Markers for Problematic Internet Use: A Telephone Survey of 2513 Adults." *CNS Spectrums* 11(10):750–55.

Black, D. W., G. Belsare, and S. Schlosser. 1999. "Clinical Features, Psychiatric Comorbidity, and Health-Related Quality of Life in Persons Reporting Compulsive Computer Use Behavior." *Journal of Clinical Psychiatry* 60(12):839–44.

Greenfield, D. N., and R. A. Davis. 2002. "Lost in Cyberspace: The Web @ Work." *Cyberpsychology and Behavior* 5(4):347–53.

Nielsen//NetRatings Web site. Available at http://www.netratings.com/pr/pr_060314.pdf. Accessed September 1, 2006.

Recupero, P., and S. E. Rainey. 2006. "Forensic Aspects of E-therapy." *Journal of Clinical Psychiatry* 67(9):1435–40.

Shapira, N. A., T. D. Goldsmith, P. E. Keck, U. M. Khosla, and S. L. McElroy. 2000. "Psychiatric Features of Individuals with Problematic Internet Use." *Journal of Affective Disorders* 57:267–72.

Young, K. S. 1998. *Caught in the Net: How to Recognize the Signs of Internet Addiction—and a Winning Strategy for Recovery.* New York: John Wiley.

ACKNOWLEDGMENTS

Many individuals contributed generously of their time, energy, and talent to bring this book to fruition. In particular, I am indebted to Dr. Donald Black for his meticulous reading of the manuscript and many helpful suggestions. I am also very grateful to Steve Rushton, Nona Gamel, Dr. Larry Koran, and my editors, Naomi Schneider, Marilyn Schwartz, and Elizabeth Berg, for their enthusiasm for the project. Above all, however, I thank my patients: they teach me something every day.

INDEX

Text:	10/15 Janson
Display:	Janson
Compositor:	Binghamton Valley Composition
Printer and binder:	Maple-Vail Manufacturing Group